The Effect of Diet on Cardiovascular Disease, Heart Disease and Blood Vessels

The Effect of Diet on Cardiovascular Disease, Heart Disease and Blood Vessels

Editor

Hayato Tada

MDPI • Basel • Beijing • Wuhan • Barcelona • Belgrade • Manchester • Tokyo • Cluj • Tianjin

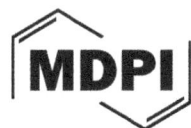

Editor
Hayato Tada
Kanazawa University
Graduate School of Medical Sciences
Japan

Editorial Office
MDPI
St. Alban-Anlage 66
4052 Basel, Switzerland

This is a reprint of articles from the Special Issue published online in the open access journal *Nutrients* (ISSN 2072-6643) (available at: https://www.mdpi.com/journal/nutrients/special_issues/cardiovascular_heart_vessels).

For citation purposes, cite each article independently as indicated on the article page online and as indicated below:

LastName, A.A.; LastName, B.B.; LastName, C.C. Article Title. *Journal Name* **Year**, *Volume Number*, Page Range.

ISBN 978-3-0365-4359-8 (Hbk)
ISBN 978-3-0365-4360-4 (PDF)

© 2022 by the authors. Articles in this book are Open Access and distributed under the Creative Commons Attribution (CC BY) license, which allows users to download, copy and build upon published articles, as long as the author and publisher are properly credited, which ensures maximum dissemination and a wider impact of our publications.

The book as a whole is distributed by MDPI under the terms and conditions of the Creative Commons license CC BY-NC-ND.

Contents

Hayato Tada, Masayuki Takamura and Masa-aki Kawashiri
The Effect of Diet on Cardiovascular Disease, Heart Disease, and Blood Vessels
Reprinted from: *Nutrients* **2022**, *14*, 246, doi:10.3390/nu14020246 1

Tetsuo Nishikawa, Yoshihiro Tanaka, Hayato Tada, Toyonobu Tsuda, Takeshi Kato, Soichiro Usui, Kenji Sakata, Kenshi Hayashi, Masa-aki Kawashiri, Atsushi Hashiba and Masayuki Takamura
Association between Cardiovascular Health and Incident Atrial Fibrillation in the General Japanese Population Aged ≥40 Years
Reprinted from: *Nutrients* **2021**, *13*, 3201, doi:10.3390/nu13093201 5

Peter E. Levanovich, Charles S. Chung, Dragana Komnenov and Noreen F. Rossi
Fructose plus High-Salt Diet in Early Life Results in Salt-Sensitive Cardiovascular Changes in Mature Male Sprague Dawley Rats
Reprinted from: *Nutrients* **2021**, *13*, 3129, doi:10.3390/nu13093129 15

Takuya Iino, Ryuji Toh, Manabu Nagao, Masakazu Shinohara, Amane Harada, Katsuhiro Murakami, Yasuhiro Irino, Makoto Nishimori, Sachiko Yoshikawa, Yutaro Seto, Tatsuro Ishida and Ken-ichi Hirata
Effects of Elaidic Acid on HDL Cholesterol Uptake Capacity
Reprinted from: *Nutrients* **2021**, *13*, 3112, doi:10.3390/nu13093112 33

Masahiro Shiozawa, Hidehiro Kaneko, Hidetaka Itoh, Kojiro Morita, Akira Okada, Satoshi Matsuoka, Hiroyuki Kiriyama, Tatsuya Kamon, Katsuhito Fujiu, Nobuaki Michihata, Taisuke Jo, Norifumi Takeda, Hiroyuki Morita, Sunao Nakamura, Koichi Node, Hideo Yasunaga and Issei Komuro
Association of Body Mass Index with Ischemic and Hemorrhagic Stroke
Reprinted from: *Nutrients* **2021**, *13*, 2343, doi:10.3390/nu13072343 47

Gustavo Henrique Ferreira Gonçalinho, Geni Rodrigues Sampaio, Rosana Aparecida Manólio Soares-Freitas and Nágila Raquel Teixeira Damasceno
Omega-3 Fatty Acids in Erythrocyte Membranes as Predictors of Lower Cardiovascular Risk in Adults without Previous Cardiovascular Events
Reprinted from: *Nutrients* **2021**, *13*, 1919, doi:10.3390/nu13061919 61

May Nasser Bin-Jumah, Sadaf Jamal Gilani, Salman Hosawi, Fahad A. Al-Abbasi, Mustafa Zeyadi, Syed Sarim Imam, Sultan Alshehri, Mohammed M Ghoneim, Muhammad Shahid Nadeem and Imran Kazmi
Pathobiological Relationship of Excessive Dietary Intake of Choline/L-Carnitine: A TMAO Precursor-Associated Aggravation in Heart Failure in Sarcopenic Patients
Reprinted from: *Nutrients* **2021**, *13*, 3453, doi:10.3390/nu13103453 75

Lan Jiang, Jinyu Wang, Ke Xiong, Lei Xu, Bo Zhang and Aiguo Ma
Intake of Fish and Marine n-3 Polyunsaturated Fatty Acids and Risk of Cardiovascular Disease Mortality: A Meta-Analysis of Prospective Cohort Studies
Reprinted from: *Nutrients* **2021**, *13*, 2342, doi:10.3390/nu13072342 87

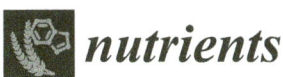

Editorial

The Effect of Diet on Cardiovascular Disease, Heart Disease, and Blood Vessels

Hayato Tada *, Masayuki Takamura and Masa-aki Kawashiri

Department of Cardiovascular Medicine, Graduate School of Medical Sciences, Kanazawa University, Kanazawa 920-1192, Japan; masayuki.takamura@gmail.com (M.T.); mk@med.kanazawa-u.ac.jp (M.-a.K.)
* Correspondence: ht240z@sa3.so-net.ne.jp; Tel.: +81-76-265-2000 (ext. 2251)

Citation: Tada, H.; Takamura, M.; Kawashiri, M.-a. The Effect of Diet on Cardiovascular Disease, Heart Disease, and Blood Vessels. *Nutrients* 2022, 14, 246. https://doi.org/10.3390/nu14020246

Received: 29 December 2021
Accepted: 29 December 2021
Published: 7 January 2022

Publisher's Note: MDPI stays neutral with regard to jurisdictional claims in published maps and institutional affiliations.

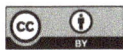

Copyright: © 2022 by the authors. Licensee MDPI, Basel, Switzerland. This article is an open access article distributed under the terms and conditions of the Creative Commons Attribution (CC BY) license (https:// creativecommons.org/licenses/by/ 4.0/).

The Effect of Diet on Cardiovascular Disease, Heart Disease, and Blood Vessels

Cardiovascular disease (CVD), including coronary artery disease, heart disease, arrhythmias, and other types of vascular diseases, are one of the leading causes of death across the world [1]. It is estimated that approximately half of the variabilities of CVD appear to be attributed to genetics [2,3]. In other words, the other half of them have been attributed to acquired factors, including diet. It is of note that even a genetic predisposition to CVD can be canceled out by a healthy lifestyle [4]. In this regard, it is important to acknowledge that acquired factors, including diet, are causally associated with CVD. Based on these facts, important papers are presented in this Special Issue entitled "The Effect of Diet on Cardiovascular Disease, Heart Disease, and Blood Vessels".

Omega-3 Polyunsaturated Fatty Acids (n-3 PUFA) and CVD

It has been suggested that our diet has a great impact on our physical function and body metabolism. Among numerous nutrients, a lot of attention has been paid to omega-3 polyunsaturated fatty acids (n-3 PUFA) that can be found in fish oil. They play important roles in various cellular functions, including signaling, cell membrane fluidity, and structural maintenance. They also regulate inflammatory processes that lead to the development of CVD. Epidemiological studies have suggested that the intake of n-3 PUFA appears to have cardioprotective effects [5,6]. Furthermore, several randomized controlled trials have suggested that supplementation on top of statins can further reduce cardiovascular risk [7,8]. The beneficial effect of n-3 PUFA has been attributed to the lowering of serum triglyceride levels; however, there appear to be other "pleiotropic" effects beyond triglycerides. Gonçalinho et al. identified one of the potential cardioprotective properties of n-3 PUFA [9]. They investigated the association between n-3 PUFA within erythrocyte membranes and established cardiovascular risk factors and found that n-3 PUFA in erythrocyte membranes are independent predictors of cardiovascular risk, comprised of multiple elements that are associated with CVD. This study suggests that n-3 PUFA contributes not only to the reduction of serum triglyceride levels but also to the modification of classical cardiovascular risk factors, such as hypertension and hyperglycemia. On the other hand, Jiang et al. nicely summarized a meta-analysis of prospective cohort studies that investigated if fish and n-3 PUFA intake are associated with reduced CVD risk [10]. It is important to note that they performed independent meta-analyses on fish intake and n-3 PUFA intake and found that both were significantly associated with reduced CVD risk. Finally, they concluded that 20 g of fish intake or 80 mg of n-3 PUFA intake per day was associated with a 4% reduction in CVD-related mortality. This study clearly suggests that the cardioprotective effect of fish intake appears to be mostly attributed to n-3 PUFA. In addition, their dose-dependent association supports the notion that the amount of intake and their serum levels are important contributors to the cardioprotective effects of n-3 PUFA supplementation. Accordingly, it may be reasonable to think about the baseline dietary pattern and serum n-3 PUFA levels of patients when considering endorsing the intake of fish or n-3 PUFA and the quantity to be taken.

On the other hand, the intake of trans fatty acids (TFA) has been associated with dyslipidemia, type 2 diabetes, CVD, and all-cause mortality [11]. As such, dietary guidelines are now recommending the non-consumption of TFAs. There are studies suggesting that TFAs are associated with dyslipidemia, type 2 diabetes, and other cardiometabolic disorders; however, Iino et al. carried out a unique study focusing on the HDL cholesterol uptake capacity. Despite the fact that statins (which can reduce LDL cholesterol) are associated with reduced CVD risk, we are still facing the reality of the so-called "residual risk" of statins [12]. There are a number of biomarkers that have been identified as such residual risk factors, including triglycerides, lipoprotein (a) (Lp(a)), and inflammation [13–15]. However, recent studies have suggested that the function of HDL, rather than HDL cholesterol, appears to be one of the most important residual risks for CVD [16]. Among the many functions of HDL, reverse cholesterol transport, also known as HDL cholesterol uptake, is the most important function in the field of preventive cardiology. In this Special Issue, they used s unique strategy for the measurement of HDL cholesterol uptake capacity in humans and found that elaidic acid, which is one of the TFAs, was associated with the inhibition of HDL cholesterol uptake and the maturation of HDL. This is strong evidence of the fact that fatty acids are involved in an important process of the development of atherosclerosis; therefore, it should be quite reasonable to accept it as a biomarker or even a source of cardioprotection.

Salt Intake and CVD

There is no doubt that hypertension is one of the leading causes of CVD. There is much evidence to support this assertion, including epidemiological studies, animal models, and randomized controlled trials [1]. Among several important factors that contribute to hypertension, the intake of salt is evidently an important one. We know that a higher intake of salt is associated with a higher risk of hypertension, and reducing one's salt intake can protect against the development of hypertension. However, there are also several important sensitivity factors associated with salt intake and the development of hypertension, including genetic factors and acquired factors, such as dietary habits other than salt intake. In this Special Issue, Levanovich et al. performed an interesting experiment using rats, showing that the consumption of 20% fructose during adolescence predisposes to salt-sensitive hypertension [17]. Importantly, they also suggested that dietary fructose intake plus a high-salt diet during this early phase leads to vascular stiffening and left ventricular diastolic dysfunction, which are both highly associated with heart failure. The underlying mechanisms are still unclear; however, it is now clear that our diet affects hypertension as well as the risk of heart failure.

Gut Microbiota and CVD

Recent studies have suggested that the gut microbiota is associated with a variety of diseases, including CVD. Although they are also affected by some genetic factors, the main factor contributing to our microbiota should be our diet. In this Special Issue, Bin-Jumah et al. nicely summarized recent findings on this matter [18]. Investigations have indicated that the gut microbiota is involved in the pathogenesis of CVD and can be considered as one of its causative factors. The gut microbiota appears to have multiple functions in humans, including energy production, maintaining intestinal homeostasis, enhancing the absorption of drugs, immune responses, defense from pathogens, and the production of microbial products, such as vitamin K, nitric oxide, trimethylamine-N-oxide (TMAO), and lipopolysaccharides. Among these properties, Bin-Jumah et al. summarized the association between TMAO and heart failure and showed that TMAO, a metabolite of the gut microbiota, may have interesting perspectives regarding how this particular metabolite contributes to the development of heart failure. They also suggested that the excessive intake of the choline of L-carnitine, which contains an intermediate precursor (TMA) of TMAO, may be harmful, especially among elderly people who have dysbiosis and muscle disorders.

Obesity and CVD

We know very well that obesity, which is greatly affected by our dietary habits, is also a major risk factor for CVD [1]. However, there is a huge gap between Asians and Caucasians in terms of the definition of "obesity". In addition, there is a paucity of data on this subject in the Asian population, where the average body mass index is much lower than that of the Caucasian population. In this Special Issue, Shiozawa et al. conducted analyses investigating an association between body mass index and stroke in the Japanese population using large health insurance databases comprising more than two million individuals. They found that overweight and obesity were associated with a greater risk of stroke and ischemic stroke in both men and women [19]. They also found that underweight, overweight, and obesity were associated with a higher risk of hemorrhagic stroke only in men. Thus, it seems that there are some gender gaps in terms of the effects of weight on CVD risk.

Lifestyle Risk Score and CVD

Finally, there is a growing trend to comprise the "risk score" in risk assessments for any conditions, such as polygenic risk scores comprising a number of common genetic variations [20]. Given that any type of CVD is associated with multiple factors, it is reasonable that such scores perform better than any single variable or parameter. Currently, the American Heart Association is advocating for the Life's Simple 7 (LS7), which consists of 7 modifiable lifestyle behaviors and medical factors, including diet, obesity, physical activity, smoking status, blood pressure, cholesterol, and glucose level) in order to reduce the prevalence of CVD and stroke [21]. This score is quite useful because it consists of simple variables that can be obtained anywhere in the world; therefore, it can be applicable to people of all ethnicities. In this Special Issue, Nishikawa et al. investigated the association between Life's Simple 7 scores among Japanese citizens and the incidence of atrial fibrillation (AF). They found that healthy lifestyle scores were associated with lower incidence rates of AF [22]. Interestingly, this trend is more remarkable among younger generations than among older generations, clearly suggesting that interventions for lifestyle factors may be better recommended for younger individuals in whom we can expect more benefits.

Author Contributions: Conceptualization, H.T., M.T. and M.-a.K.; manuscript preparation, H.T., M.T. and M.-a.K.; review and editing, H.T., M.T. and M.-a.K. All authors have read and agreed to the published version of the manuscript.

Funding: This research received no external funding.

Conflicts of Interest: The authors declare no conflict of interest.

References

1. Virani, S.S.; Alonso, A.; Aparicio, H.J.; Benjamin, E.J.; Bittencourt, M.S.; Callaway, C.W.; Carson, A.P.; Chamberlain, A.M.; Cheng, S.; Delling, F.N.; et al. Heart disease and stroke statistics-2021 update: A report from the American heart association. *Circulation* **2021**, *143*, e254–e743. [CrossRef] [PubMed]
2. Tada, H.; Fujino, N.; Nomura, A.; Nakanishi, C.; Hayashi, K.; Takamura, M.; Kawashiri, M.A. Personalized medicine for cardiovascular diseases. *J. Hum. Genet.* **2021**, *66*, 67–74. [CrossRef] [PubMed]
3. Tada, H.; Fujino, N.; Hayashi, K.; Kawashiri, M.A.; Takamura, M. Human genetics and its impact on cardiovascular disease. *J. Cardiol.* **2022**, *79*, 233–239. [CrossRef]
4. Khera, A.V.; Emdin, C.A.; Drake, I.; Natarajan, P.; Bick, A.G.; Cook, N.R.; Chasman, D.I.; Baber, U.; Mehran, R.; Rader, D.J.; et al. Genetic risk, adherence to a healthy lifestyle, and coronary disease. *N. Engl. J. Med.* **2016**, *375*, 2349–2358. [CrossRef]
5. Iso, H.; Kobayashi, M.; Ishihara, J.; Sasaki, S.; Okada, K.; Kita, Y.; Kokubo, Y.; Tsugane, S.; JPHC Study Group. Intake of fish and n3 fatty acids and risk of coronary heart disease among Japanese: The Japan public health center-based (JPHC) study cohort I. *Circulation* **2006**, *113*, 195–202. [CrossRef] [PubMed]
6. Amano, T.; Matsubara, T.; Uetani, T.; Kato, M.; Kato, B.; Yoshida, T.; Harada, K.; Kumagai, S.; Kunimura, A.; Shinbo, Y.; et al. Impact of omega-3 polyunsaturated fatty acids on coronary plaque instability: An integrated backscatter intravascular ultrasound study. *Atherosclerosis* **2011**, *218*, 110–116. [CrossRef] [PubMed]

7. Yokoyama, M.; Origasa, H.; Matsuzaki, M.; Matsuzawa, Y.; Saito, Y.; Ishikawa, Y.; Oikawa, S.; Sasaki, J.; Hishida, H.; Itakura, H.; et al. Effects of eicosapentaenoic acid on major coronary events in hypercholesterolaemic patients (JELIS): A randomised open-label, blinded endpoint analysis. *Lancet* **2007**, *369*, 1090–1098. [CrossRef]
8. Bhatt, D.L.; Steg, P.G.; Miller, M.; Brinton, E.A.; Jacobson, T.A.; Ketchum, S.B.; Doyle, R.T., Jr.; Juliano, R.A.; Jiao, L.; Granowitz, C.; et al. Cardiovascular risk reduction with icosapent ethyl for hypertriglyceridemia. *N. Engl. J. Med.* **2019**, *380*, 11–22. [CrossRef] [PubMed]
9. Gonçalinho, G.H.F.; Sampaio, G.R.; Soares-Freitas, R.A.M.; Damasceno, N.R.T. Omega-3 Fatty acids in erythrocyte membranes as predictors of lower cardiovascular risk in adults without previous cardiovascular events. *Nutrients* **2021**, *13*, 1919. [CrossRef] [PubMed]
10. Jiang, L.; Wang, J.; Xiong, K.; Xu, L.; Zhang, B.; Ma, A. Intake of fish and marine n-3 polyunsaturated fatty acids and risk of cardiovascular disease mortality: A meta-analysis of prospective cohort studies. *Nutrients* **2021**, *13*, 2342. [CrossRef]
11. Islam, M.A.; Amin, M.N.; Siddiqui, S.A.; Hossain, M.P.; Sultana, F.; Kabir, M.R. Trans fatty acids and lipid profile: A serious risk factor to cardiovascular disease, cancer and diabetes. *Diabetes Metab. Syndr.* **2019**, *13*, 1643–1647. [CrossRef]
12. Iino, T.; Toh, R.; Nagao, M.; Shinohara, M.; Harada, A.; Murakami, K.; Irino, Y.; Nishimori, M.; Yoshikawa, S.; Seto, Y.; et al. Effects of elaidic acid on HDL cholesterol uptake capacity. *Nutrients* **2021**, *13*, 3112. [CrossRef]
13. Tada, H.; Kawashiri, M.A. Genetic variations, triglycerides, and atherosclerotic disease. *J. Atheroscler. Thromb.* **2019**, *26*, 128–131. [CrossRef] [PubMed]
14. Tada, H.; Nomura, A.; Yoshimura, K.; Itoh, H.; Komuro, I.; Yamagishi, M.; Takamura, M.; Kawashiri, M.A. Fasting and non-fasting triglycerides and risk of cardiovascular events in diabetic patients under statin therapy. *Circ. J.* **2020**, *84*, 509–515. [CrossRef] [PubMed]
15. Tada, H.; Takamura, M.; Kawashiri, M.A. Lipoprotein(a) as an old and new causal risk factor of atherosclerotic cardiovascular disease. *J. Atheroscler. Thromb.* **2019**, *26*, 583–591. [CrossRef] [PubMed]
16. Khera, A.V.; Cuchel, M.; de la Llera-Moya, M.; Rodrigues, A.; Burke, M.F.; Jafri, K.; French, B.C.; Phillips, J.A.; Mucksavage, M.L.; Wilensky, R.L.; et al. Cholesterol efflux capacity, high-density lipoprotein function, and atherosclerosis. *N. Engl. J. Med.* **2011**, *364*, 127–135. [CrossRef] [PubMed]
17. Levanovich, P.E.; Chung, C.S.; Komnenov, D.; Rossi, N.F. Fructose plus high-salt diet in early life results in salt-sensitive cardiovascular changes in mature male sprague dawley rats. *Nutrients* **2021**, *13*, 3129. [CrossRef] [PubMed]
18. Bin-Jumah, M.N.; Gilani, S.J.; Hosawi, S.; Al-Abbasi, F.A.; Zeyadi, M.; Imam, S.S.; Alshehri, S.; Ghoneim, M.M.; Nadeem, M.S.; Kazmi, I. Pathobiological relationship of excessive dietary intake of choline/L-carnitine: A TMAO precursor-associated aggravation in heart failure in sarcopenic patients. *Nutrients* **2021**, *13*, 3453. [CrossRef]
19. Shiozawa, M.; Kaneko, H.; Itoh, H.; Morita, K.; Okada, A.; Matsuoka, S.; Kiriyama, H.; Kamon, T.; Fujiu, K.; Michihata, N.; et al. Association of body mass index with ischemic and hemorrhagic stroke. *Nutrients* **2021**, *13*, 2343. [CrossRef]
20. Tada, H.; Melander, O.; Louie, J.Z.; Catanese, J.J.; Rowland, C.M.; Devlin, J.J.; Kathiresan, S.; Shiffman, D. Risk prediction by genetic risk scores for coronary heart disease is independent of self-reported family history. *Eur. Heart. J.* **2016**, *37*, 561–567. [CrossRef]
21. Lloyd-Jones, D.M.; Hong, Y.; Labarthe, D.; Mozaffarian, D.; Appel, L.J.; Van Horn, L.; Greenlund, K.; Daniels, S.; Nichol, G.; Tomaselli, G.F.; et al. Defining and setting national goals for cardiovascular health promotion and disease reduction: The American heart association's strategic impact goal through 2020 and beyond. *Circulation* **2010**, *121*, 586–613. [CrossRef] [PubMed]
22. Nishikawa, T.; Tanaka, Y.; Tada, H.; Tsuda, T.; Kato, T.; Usui, S.; Sakata, K.; Hayashi, K.; Kawashiri, M.A.; Hashiba, A.; et al. Association between cardiovascular health and incident atrial fibrillation in the general Japanese population aged 40 years. *Nutrients* **2021**, *13*, 3201. [CrossRef] [PubMed]

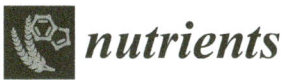

Article

Association between Cardiovascular Health and Incident Atrial Fibrillation in the General Japanese Population Aged ≥40 Years

Tetsuo Nishikawa [1,†], Yoshihiro Tanaka [2,3,†], Hayato Tada [1,*], Toyonobu Tsuda [1], Takeshi Kato [1], Soichiro Usui [1], Kenji Sakata [1], Kenshi Hayashi [1], Masa-aki Kawashiri [1], Atsushi Hashiba [4] and Masayuki Takamura [1]

[1] Department of Cardiovascular Medicine, Kanazawa University Graduate School of Medical Sciences, Kanazawa 920-8641, Japan; tetsunishi25@gmail.com (T.N.); ttsuda0329@yahoo.co.jp (T.T.); takeshikato@mac.com (T.K.); usuiso@staff.kanazawa-u.ac.jp (S.U.); kenjis@yu.incl.ne.jp (K.S.); kenshi@med.kanazawa-u.ac.jp (K.H.); mk@med.kanazawa-u.ac.jp (M.-a.K.); masayuki.takamura@gmail.com (M.T.)
[2] Department of Preventive Medicine, Northwestern University Feinberg School of Medicine, Chicago, IL 60611, USA; y.tanaka@northwestern.edu
[3] Center for Arrhythmia Research, Northwestern University Feinberg School of Medicine, Chicago, IL 60611, USA
[4] Kanazawa Medical Association, Kanazawa 920-0912, Japan; hashiba.atsushi.kanazawa@gmail.com
* Correspondence: ht240z@sa3.so-net.ne.jp; Tel.: +81-76-265-2000 (ext. 2251)
† These authors contributed equally to this work.

Abstract: This study explores the association between lifestyle behavior and incident atrial fibrillation (AF) in the general Japanese population. Japanese residents aged ≥40 years undergoing a national health checkup in Kanazawa City were included. We hypothesized that better lifestyle behavior is associated with lower incidence of AF. Lifestyle behavior was evaluated by the total cardiovascular health (CVH) score (0 = poor to 14 = ideal), calculated as the sum of the individual scores on seven modifiable risk factors: smoking status, physical activity, obesity, patterns of eating schedule, blood pressure, total cholesterol, and blood glucose. The association between CVH and incident AF was assessed, adjusting for other factors. A total of 37,523 participants (mean age 72.3 ± 9.6 years, 36.8% men, and mean total CVH score 9 ± 1) were analyzed. During the median follow-up period of 5 years, 703 cases of incident AF were observed. Using a low CVH score as a reference, the upper group (ideal CVH group) had a significantly lower risk of incident AF (hazard ratio [HR] = 0.79, 95% confidence interval 0.65–0.96, p = 0.02), especially among those aged <75 years (HR = 0.68, 95% confidence interval 0.49–0.94, p = 0.02). Thus, ideal CVH is independently associated with a lower risk for incident AF, particularly in younger Japanese individuals (<75 years).

Keywords: cardiovascular health; atrial fibrillation; Japanese

1. Introduction

Atrial fibrillation (AF) is the most common arrhythmia in the world, with an incidence that increases annually, and it is associated with a rising risk of stroke, cardiovascular morbidity, physical disability, dementia, and mortality [1–3]. In Japan, the number of patients who will develop AF by 2030 is estimated to be greater than 1 million [4]. Therefore, more studies focusing on preventative approaches to AF are warranted. Established risk factors of AF include aging, hypertension, obesity, smoking, cardiac disease (valvular disease, cardiomyopathy, coronary artery disease, and heart failure), hyperthyroidism, and diabetes mellitus. It is noteworthy that these factors are also known to lead to other cardiovascular diseases [5,6]. Among them, lifestyle behaviors are attracting more attention as modifiable risk factors of AF and other cardiovascular diseases. The American Heart Association already advocates the Life's Simple 7 (LS7), which consists of seven modifiable lifestyle behaviors and medical factors (diet, obesity, physical activity, smoking status, blood pressure, total cholesterol, and blood glucose) to improve cardiovascular health (CVH) and reduce

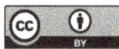

cardiovascular disease and stroke [7]. Using the LS7 metrics, previous studies revealed that ideal CVH is associated with a reduced risk of AF in Western populations [5,8,9]. Moreover, a cohort study revealed that an intervention for CVH such as reduction in body weight improved arrhythmia-free survival after ablation of AF in the Australian population [10]. However, insufficient data exist regarding this issue in the Asian population, especially among Japanese individuals. Only one study showed abdominal obesity and habitual behaviors, such as smoking status, alcohol intake, and physical activity, to be associated with an increased incidence of AF [11]. Thus, we conducted this study to explore the association between CVH and incident AF in the general Japanese population under the hypothesis that better lifestyle behavior is associated with lower incidence of AF, using large samples (>30,000) of the Japanese-specific health checkups in Kanazawa City.

2. Materials and Methods

We included patients who had undergone Japanese-specific health checkups in Kanazawa City, which is a strategy of the Japanese government to provide an early screen for, diagnose, and treat the metabolic syndrome that started in 2008. All general residents in Kanazawa City aged 40 years or older were eligible. The participants completed questionnaires about medical history, medications, and lifestyles. Examinations included anthropometric measurements, physical examinations, blood tests, urine dipstick tests, and resting 12-lead electrocardiogram (ECG).

2.1. Study Participants

Eligible participants were Japanese residents aged ≥40 years who had undergone 12-lead ECG at the Japanese-specific health checkups in Kanazawa City in 2013 (n = 47,551; Figure 1). We excluded participants with missing baseline characteristics, those who did not complete a follow-up examination at least once during a 5-year follow-up period, those with AF detected at the baseline ECG, and those without adequate follow-up (n = 10,028). An event was defined as a new onset of AF diagnosed by automatic analysis of ECG based on the Minnesota code (8-3) during the follow-up period. Results of all automatically coded ECGs were confirmed by experienced physicians for health checkups.

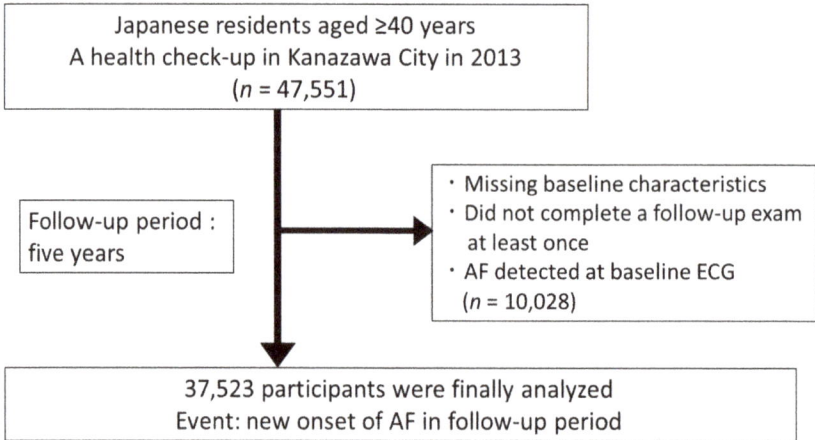

Figure 1. Study flow chart. Eligible participants were Japanese residents aged ≥40 years who had undergone 12-lead electrocardiogram (ECG) during a Japanese-specific health checkup in Kanazawa City in 2013 (n = 47,551). We excluded participants with missing baseline characteristics, those who did not complete a follow-up examination at least once during the 5-year follow-up period, those with AF detected at the baseline ECG, and those without adequate follow-up (n = 10,028). An event was defined as a new onset of AF diagnosed by automatic analysis of ECG based on the Minnesota code (8-3) during the follow-up period.

2.2. CVH Score

We defined the CVH score to evaluate seven modifiable risk factors following LS7 (Figure 2). The total CVH score ranged from 0 (poor) to 14 (ideal) and was calculated as the sum of the individual scores on seven modifiable risk factors (patterns of eating schedule, obesity, physical activity, smoking status, blood pressure, total cholesterol, and blood glucose). Patterns of eating schedule was scored by three answers from the questionnaire (eating faster than ordinary, eating dinner within 2 h before sleep at least three times per week, and eating snacks after dinner at least three times per week). We scored 2 points (ideal) if answers applied to none of the three questions, 0 points (poor) if the answers applied to all three questions, and 1 point if the answers applied to one or two questions. Obesity was scored by body mass index (BMI). We scored 2 points if BMI was less than 25 kg/m^2, 0 points if BMI was 30 kg/m^2 or greater, and 1point if BMI was between 25 and 29.9 kg/m^2. Physical activity was scored by three answers from the questionnaire (exercising for 30 min per day at least two times per week over 1 year, walking or exercising 1 h per day on a daily basis, walking faster than people of the same sex and age). We scored 2 points (ideal) if the answers applied to all three questions, 0 points (poor) if the answers applied to none of the questions, and 1 point if the answers applied to one or two questions. Smoking status was scored as 2 points for noncurrent smoker and 0 points for current smoker. Blood pressure was scored as 2 points if systolic blood pressure (SBP) was <120 mmHg and diastolic blood pressure (DBP) was <80 mmHg without antihypertensive drugs. It was scored as 0 points if SBP was greater than or equal to 140 mmHg or DBP was greater than or equal to 90 mmHg, and 1 point if it was not applied to either condition. Total cholesterol (TC) was scored as 2 points if the TC was <200 mg/dL without lipid-lowering drugs, 0 points if the TC was greater than or equal to 240 mg/dL, and 1 point if it was not applied to either condition. Blood glucose was scored as 2 points if the fasting blood glucose (FBG) was less than 100 mg/dL without oral hyperglycemic drugs or insulin, 0 points if the FBG was greater than or equal to 126 mg/dL, and 1 point if it was not applied to either condition.

Cardiovascular health (CVH) score	Ideal (2 points)	Intermediate (1 point)	Poor (0 points)
Patterns of Eating Schedule	• Eating faster than the ordinary • Eating dinner within 2 hours before sleep at least three times a week • Eating snacks after dinner at least three times a week		
	Apply to no conditions	Apply to one or two conditions	Apply to all three conditions
Obesity	BMI <25 kg/m^2	BMI 25–29.9 kg/m^2	BMI ≥30 kg/m^2
Physical activity	• Exercise for 30 minutes a day at least two times a week over 1 year • Walking or exercise 1 hour a day on a daily basis • Walking faster than people of the same sex and age		
	Apply to all three conditions	Apply to one or two conditions	Apply to no conditions
Smoking status	Non–current smoker	–	Current smoker
Blood pressure SBP: systolic blood pressure DBP: diastolic blood pressure	SBP <120 mmHg and DBP <80 mmHg, without antihypertensive drugs	SBP 120–139 mmHg, DBP 80–89 mmHg, or better control with antihypertensive drugs	SBP ≥140 mmHg or DBP ≥90 mmHg
Total cholesterol TC: total cholesterol	TC <200 mg/dL without lipid–lowering drugs	TC 200–239 mg/dL or better control with lipid–lowering drugs	TC ≥240 mg/dL
Blood glucose FBG: fasting blood glucose	FBG <100 mg/dL without oral hypoglycemic drugs or insulin	FBG 100–125 mg/dL or better control with oral hypoglycemic drugs or insulin	FBG ≥126 mg/dL

Figure 2. Cardiovascular health (CVH) scoring. The CVH score included seven modifiable components (patterns of eating schedule, obesity, physical activity, smoking status, blood pressure, total cholesterol, and blood glucose). We referred to the data of health checkups from questionnaires, anthropometric measurements, and blood tests. BMI, body mass index.

2.3. Statistical Analysis

Continuous variables were expressed as mean ± standard deviation, and categorical variables were expressed as number and percentage. Differences in the baseline characteristics were compared using Student's *t*-test for parametric data and the Mann–Whitney *U* test for nonparametric data. Categorical variables were compared using the chi-square or Fisher's exact tests. Cox proportional hazard models were used to identify independent associations with the outcomes.

A *p*-value of <0.05 was considered statistically significant. We used R statistical software for all analyses.

2.4. Ethical Considerations

The Ethics Committee of Kanazawa Medical Association (16000003) and Kanazawa University (2019-223) approved this study. The research was conducted in accordance with the Declaration of Helsinki (2008) by the World Medical Association. All procedures were performed in accordance with the ethical standards of the responsible committee on human experimentation (institutional and national) and with the Helsinki Declaration of 1975 (as revised in 2008).

3. Results

3.1. Study Characteristics

Table 1 shows the basic characteristics of this study population. A total of 37,523 participants (mean age 72.3 ± 9.6 years, 36.8% men, and mean total CVH score 9 ± 1) were finally analyzed. During the median follow-up period of 5 years (interquartile range 3.99–5.02), 703 cases of incident AF were observed. There were significant differences in age, sex, SBP, BMI, history of coronary artery disease, stroke, alcohol intake, and estimated glomerular filtration rate (eGFR) between the AF group and the non-AF group. The AF group was significantly older, had a significantly higher proportion of men, and had a significantly greater BMI than the non-AF group. The AF group had a more frequent history of heart disease and stroke. The AF group had a more frequent regular alcohol intake and lower eGFR.

Table 1. Basic characteristics of the study population. Regular alcohol intake meant drinking every day. SBP, systolic blood pressure; DBP, diastolic blood pressure; BMI, body mass index; eGFR, estimated glomerular filtration rate.

Variables	Total N = 37,523	AF (−) n = 36,820	AF (+) n = 703	*p*-Value
Age, years	72.3 (9.6)	72.2 (9.6)	77.3 (8.0)	<0.01
Male, n (%)	13,799 (37%)	13,401 (36%)	398 (57%)	<0.01
SBP, mmHg	128 (15)	128 (15)	130 (15)	<0.01
DBP, mmHg	73 (10)	73 (10)	74 (10)	0.37
BMI, kg/m^2	22.9 (3.3)	22.8 (3.3)	23.6 (3.4)	<0.01
Smoking, n (%)	3528 (9.4%)	3458 (9.4%)	70 (10%)	0.66
Total cholesterol, mg/dL	196 (33)	196 (33)	185 (31)	<0.01
Fasting blood glucose, mg/dL	104 (29)	104 (29)	108 (31)	<0.01
eGFR, mL/min/1.73 m^2	71.7 (17.3)	71.8 (17.3)	66.0 (17.2)	<0.01
Coronary artery disease, n (%)	4323 (12%)	4013 (11%)	220 (31%)	<0.01
Stroke, n (%)	2583 (7%)	2494 (7%)	89 (13%)	<0.01
Regular alcohol intake, n (%)	8457 (23%)	8285 (22%)	212 (30%)	<0.01
Total cardiovascular health score	9 (8–10)	9 (8–10)	9 (8–10)	<0.01
Smoking	2 (2–2)	2 (2–2)	2 (2–2)	<0.01
Physical activity	1 (1–1)	1 (1–1)	1 (0–1)	<0.01
Obesity	2 (1–2)	2 (1–2)	2 (1–2)	<0.01
Patterns of eating schedule	1 (1–2)	1 (1–2)	1 (1–2)	<0.01
Blood pressure	1 (1–1)	1 (1–1)	1 (1–1)	0.13
Total cholesterol	1 (1–1)	1 (1–1)	1 (1–2)	0.25
Blood glucose	2 (2–2)	2 (2–2)	2 (2–2)	0.64

3.2. Total CVH Score

Total CVH scores were normally distributed and ranged from 1 to 14, with a mean value of 9.25 ± 1.66. We classified a total CVH score of 1–9 as the poor CVH group (N = 20,177), a total CVH score of 10 as the intermediate CVH group (N = 8819), and a total CVH score of 11–14 as the ideal CVH group (N = 8527), based on the number of individuals according to the distribution. (Figure 3A). We observed 420, 126, and 157 AF incidents among the poor (85,230 person-years), intermediate (37,534 person-years), and ideal (38,349 person-years) groups, respectively (Figure 3B). The incident rate of AF per 1000 was 4.9, 4.1, and 3.6 in the poor, intermediate, and ideal groups, respectively. Compared with the poor CVH group, the ideal CVH group had a significantly lower risk for incident AF (chi-squared test, $p = 0.0002$).

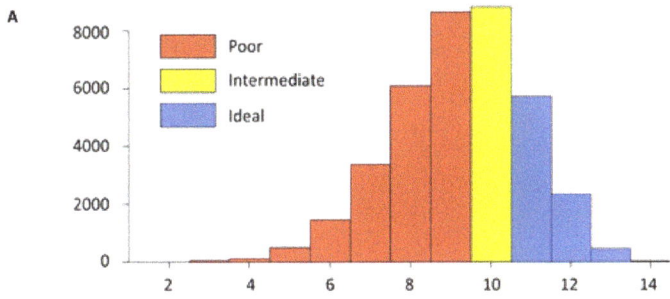

Figure 3. (**A**) Histogram of total cardiovascular health (CVH) score. The horizontal axis shows the total CVH score, and the vertical axis shows the number of participants. We classified a total CVH score of 1–9 as the poor CVH group (red), a total CVH score of 10 as the intermediate CVH group (yellow), and a total CVH score of 11–14 as the ideal CVH group (blue). (**B**) Incident rate of atrial fibrillation by three groups of total CVH scores.

3.3. Association between CVH and Incident AF

Using the poor CVH group as a reference, the ideal CVH group had a significantly lower risk of incident AF (hazard ratio (HR) = 0.75, 95% confidence interval 0.61–0.92, $p = 0.005$), in model 1, adjusting for age gender, and regular alcohol intake (Table 2). Likewise, the ideal CVH group had a significantly lower risk of incident AF compared with the poor CVH group (HR = 0.79, 95% confidence interval 0.65–0.96, $p = 0.02$) in model 2, adjusting for age, gender, history of heart disease, history of stroke, alcohol intake, eGFR. In model 2, we also observed other factors that were significantly associated with increased or decreased risk for AF, including age (HR = 1.07, 95% confidence interval 1.06–1.08, $p = 2.0 \times 10^{-16}$), female sex (HR = 0.48, 95% confidence interval 0.41–0.57, $p = 2.0 \times 10^{-16}$), no history of heart disease (HR = 0.38, 95% confidence interval 0.32–0.45, $p = 2.0 \times 10^{-16}$), no history of stroke (HR = 0.78, 95% confidence interval 0.62–0.97, $p = 0.029$), not drinking alcohol (HR = 0.76, 95% confidence interval 0.63–0.92, $p = 0.005$), and eGFR (HR = 0.99, 95% confidence interval 0.989–0.998, $p = 0.007$).

Table 2. Association between cardiovascular health (CVH) score and incident atrial fibrillation in all participants. Model 1 was adjusted for age, gender, and regular alcohol intake. Model 2 was adjusted for age, gender, history of heart disease, history of stroke, regular alcohol intake, and estimated glomerular filtration rate (eGFR). The hazard ratio of the intermediate and ideal CVH groups was calculated using the poor CVH group as a reference.

Model 1	Hazard Ratio	Lower 95% CI	Upper 95% CI	p-Value
Age	1.08	1.07	1.09	$<2 \times 10^{-16}$
Female	0.44	0.37	0.52	$<2 \times 10^{-16}$
No alcohol intake	0.82	0.67	0.99	0.04
Intermediate CVH	0.89	0.74	1.07	0.21
Ideal CVH	0.75	0.61	0.92	0.005
Model 2	Hazard ratio	Lower 95% CI	Upper 95% CI	p-Value
Age	1.07	1.06	1.08	$<2 \times 10^{-16}$
Female	0.48	0.41	0.57	$<2 \times 10^{-16}$
No history of heart disease	0.38	0.32	0.45	$<2 \times 10^{-16}$
No history of stroke	0.78	0.62	0.97	0.03
No alcohol intake	0.76	0.63	0.92	0.005
eGFR	0.994	0.989	0.998	0.006
Intermediate CVH	0.92	0.76	1.1	0.36
Ideal CVH	0.79	0.65	0.96	0.02

3.4. Subanalysis Focusing on the Younger Group (Aged <75 Years)

We also investigated whether the influence of CVH on incident AF was more profound in the younger group as compared with the older group (Table 3). We divided the younger group and elder group by age 75 years based on the following two reasons: (1) age 75 years was close to the median age in this study (Supplemental Figure S1) and (2) age 75 years or older was defined as advanced elderly in Japan. In participants aged <75 years, using the poor CVH group as a reference, the ideal CVH group had a significantly lower risk of incident AF (HR = 0.64, 95% confidence interval 0.46–0.88, $p = 0.006$) in model 1, adjusting for age, gender, and regular alcohol intake. Likewise, the ideal CVH group had a significantly lower risk of incident AF as compared with the poor CVH group (HR = 0.68, 95% confidence interval 0.49–0.94, $p = 0.02$) in model 2, adjusting for age, sex, history of heart disease, history of stroke, alcohol intake, and eGFR in the younger group. In model 2 in the younger group, we also observed other factors that had a significant difference: age (HR = 1.07, 95% confidence interval 1.04–1.10, $p = 3.7 \times 10^{-6}$), female sex (HR = 0.42, 95% confidence interval 0.32–0.57, $p = 5.2 \times 10^{-9}$), no history of heart disease (HR = 0.27, 95% confidence interval 0.20–0.35, $p = 2.0 \times 10^{-16}$), no history of stroke (HR = 0.54, 95% confidence interval 0.37–0.78, $p = 0.025$), and not drinking alcohol (HR = 0.71, 95% confidence interval 0.53–0.96, $p = 0.02$).

3.5. Subanalysis Focusing on the Older Group (Aged ≥75 Years)

In participants aged ≥75 years, there was no significant difference between the poor CVH group and the ideal CVH group (HR = 0.85, 95% confidence interval 0.66–1.10, $p = 0.21$) in model 1, adjusting for age, gender, and regular alcohol intake (Table 4). Similarly, there was no significant difference between the poor CVH group and the ideal CVH group (HR = 0.88, 95% confidence interval 0.69–1.14, $p = 0.34$) in model 2, adjusting for age, sex, history of heart disease, history of stroke, alcohol intake, and eGFR in the older group. In model 2, in the older group, we also observed other factors that were significantly different: age (HR = 1.08, 95% confidence interval 1.06–1.10, $p = 3.1 \times 10^{-13}$), female sex (HR = 0.52, 95% confidence interval 0.42–0.65, $p = 2.7 \times 10^{-9}$), no history of heart disease (HR = 0.46, 95% confidence interval 0.38–0.57, $p = 1.4 \times 10^{-13}$).

Table 3. Association between cardiovascular health (CVH) score and incident atrial fibrillation in younger participants (<75 years). Model 1 was adjusted for age, gender, and regular alcohol intake. Model 2 was adjusted for age, gender, history of heart disease, history of stroke, regular alcohol intake, and estimated glomerular filtration rate. The hazard ratio of the intermediate and ideal CVH groups was calculated using the poor CVH group as a reference.

Model 1	Hazard Ratio	Lower 95% CI	Upper 95% CI	p-Value
Age	1.09	1.06	1.11	1.9×10^{-9}
Female	0.36	0.27	0.48	1.5×10^{-12}
No alcohol intake	0.76	0.57	1.03	0.08
Intermediate CVH	0.79	0.58	1.07	0.12
Ideal CVH	0.64	0.46	0.88	0.006
Model 2	Hazard ratio	Lower 95% CI	Upper 95% CI	p-Value
Age	1.07	1.04	1.10	3.7×10^{-6}
Female	0.43	0.32	0.57	5.2×10^{-9}
No history of heart disease	0.27	0.2	0.35	$<2 \times 10^{-16}$
No history of stroke	0.54	0.37	0.78	0.001
No alcohol intake	0.71	0.53	0.96	0.03
eGFR	0.99	0.98	1.00	0.056
Intermediate CVH	0.83	0.61	1.12	0.22
Ideal CVH	0.68	0.49	0.94	0.02

Table 4. Association between cardiovascular health (CVH) score and incident atrial fibrillation in younger participants (≥75 years). Model 1 was adjusted for age, gender, and regular alcohol intake. Model 2 was adjusted for age, gender, history of heart disease, history of stroke, regular alcohol intake, and estimated glomerular filtration rate. The hazard ratio of the intermediate and ideal CVH groups was calculated using the poor CVH group as a reference.

Model 1	Hazard Ratio	Lower 95% CI	Upper 95% CI	p-Value
Age	1.09	1.07	1.11	$<2.0 \times 10^{-16}$
Female	0.49	0.4	0.61	4.0×10^{-11}
No alcohol intake	0.84	0.66	1.08	0.19
Intermediate CVH	0.97	0.77	1.22	0.79
Ideal CVH	0.85	0.66	1.10	0.21
Model 2	Hazard ratio	Lower 95% CI	Upper 95% CI	p-Value
Age	1.08	1.06	1.10	3.1×10^{-13}
Female	0.52	0.42	0.65	2.7×10^{-9}
No history of heart disease	0.46	0.38	0.57	1.4×10^{-13}
No history of stroke	0.91	0.68	1.21	0.52
No alcohol intake	0.8	0.62	1.02	0.06
eGFR	0.99	0.99	1.00	0.06
Intermediate CVH	0.99	0.79	1.25	0.95
Ideal CVH	0.88	0.69	1.14	0.34

4. Discussion

Analyzing a large dataset from the Japanese-specific health checkups in Kanazawa City, we observed the following: (1) the ideal CVH was associated with lower incident AF independently of conventional risk factors of AF, (2) an ideal CVH had a larger impact on lowering incident AF in the younger generation (aged <75 years). Our CVH score could be automatically and easily calculated from the questionnaire and measurements obtained from the health checkups. It might be helpful to enlighten participants on their risk of incident AF and encourage the modification of CVH. In observational studies, optimal CVH was associated with a lower risk of incident AF [5,8,9]. In secondary prevention, we observed less frequent AF in the group that had aggressive risk modification, such as with body weight reduction [10]. On the other hand, there were only a few studies regarding this issue in the primary prevention settings [12,13]. Moreover, all of the above studies were from Western countries.

Indeed, ideal CVH is associated with a great reduction in coronary artery disease (79% in men and 72.7% in women), for which the risk factors overlap those of AF [14,15]. Thus, according to these results, as with coronary artery disease, CVH should have a great contribution to incident AF. From the results of our study, a CVH intervention in the younger population might be effective. Therefore, further trials of CVH intervention focused on the younger population are needed. Moreover, we also found that alcohol intake was significantly associated with incident AF as previously described [16]. Accordingly, drinking restrictions should also be considered together with CVH intervention among Japanese as well.

Limitations

This study has several limitations. First, this was a retrospective study. Second, there were more female participants in the Japanese-specific health checkups in Kanazawa City, which could potentially have affected the results. This is because these health checkups were for housewives or unemployed persons instead of health checkups in their workplace. In Japan, a "regular" worker must undergo health checkups offered by their workplaces, instead of these specific health checkups. Actually, more males work regularly than females in Japan. Third, a diagnosis of AF in the health checkups depended on an ECG that was performed only once per year. Thus, we might have missed paroxysmal AF. Fourth, our definitions of eating habits and exercise were different from those of the American Heart Association's LS7. For eating habits, our definition focused on eating time and speed of eating. On the other hand, the American Heart Association's definition focused on the content of the diet. Fifth, this study assessed the participants' lifestyle at the inclusion cross-sectionally and thus did not address the effect of changes in CVH on incident AF during the follow-up period. Prospective studies with lifestyle interventions are needed to fully address this important issue in the future. Finally, this study did not assess the food composite in these health checkups. However, patterns of eating schedule have been shown to be associated with cardiovascular disease and stroke among the Japanese population [17]; thus, this element is employed in most of the health checkups in Japan. We believe that this factor can serve as a substitute for the food composite, at least among the Japanese population.

5. Conclusions

Ideal CVH is independently associated with a lower risk for incident AF, especially in the younger Japanese population (<75 years).

Supplementary Materials: The following are available online at https://www.mdpi.com/article/10.3390/nu13093201/s1. Figure S1: Histogram of age in this study. The horizontal axis shows the participants' ages, and the vertical axis shows the number of participants. The dashed line is drawn at age 75 years. The median age of this study was 72.0 years.

Author Contributions: Conceptualization, T.N., Y.T., H.T., T.K., M.-a.K., and M.T.; methodology, Y.T. and H.T.; validation, Y.T., and H.T.; formal analysis, T.N., Y.T., and H.T.; investigation, T.N., Y.T., H.T., T.T., T.K., S.U., K.S., K.H., M.-a.K., A.H., and M.T.; resources, A.H.; data curation, A.H.; writing—original draft preparation, T.N., Y.T., H.T., T.T., T.K., S.U., K.S., K.H., M.-a.K., A.H., and M.T.; writing—review and editing, T.N., Y.T., H.T., T.T., T.K., S.U., K.S., K.H., M.-a.K., A.H., and M.T.; visualization, T.N., Y.T., H.T., T.T., T.K., S.U., K.S., K.H., M.-a.K., A.H., and M.T.; supervision, H.T. and M.T.; project administration, A.H. All authors have read and agreed to the published version of the manuscript.

Funding: This research received no external funding.

Institutional Review Board Statement: The study was conducted according to the guidelines of the Declaration of Helsinki and approved by the Institutional Review Board (or Ethics Committee) of Kanazawa University (2019-223) and Kanazawa Medical Association (16000003).

Informed Consent Statement: Written informed consent has been obtained from the patients to publish this paper.

Data Availability Statement: The data presented in this study are available on request from the corresponding author. The data are not publicly available due to our regulations.

Acknowledgments: We would like to express special thanks to Yoshitaka Sakikawa (staff of Kanazawa Medical Association).

Conflicts of Interest: The authors declare no conflict of interest.

References

1. Lip, G.Y.H.; Lane, D.A. Stroke prevention in atrial fibrillation: A systematic review. *JAMA* **2015**, *313*, 1950–1962. [CrossRef] [PubMed]
2. Rienstra, M.; Lubitz, S.A.; Mahida, S.; Magnani, J.W.; Fontes, J.D.; Sinner, M.F.; Van Gelder, I.C.; Ellinor, P.T.; Benjamin, E.J. Symptoms and functional status of patients with atrial fibrillation: State of the art and future research opportunities. *Circulation* **2012**, *125*, 2933–2943. [CrossRef] [PubMed]
3. Kalantarian, S.; Stern, T.A.; Mansour, M.; Ruskin, J.N. Cognitive impairment associated with atrial fibrillation: A meta-analysis. *Ann. Intern. Med.* **2013**, *158*, 338–346. [CrossRef] [PubMed]
4. Inoue, H.; Fujiki, A.; Origasa, H.; Ogawa, S.; Okumura, K.; Kubota, I.; Aizawa, Y.; Yamashita, T.; Atarashi, H.; Horie, M.; et al. Prevalence of atrial fibrillation in the general population of Japan: An analysis based on periodic health examination. *Int. J. Cardiol.* **2009**, *137*, 102–107. [CrossRef] [PubMed]
5. Garg, P.K.; O'Neal, W.T.; Chen, L.Y.; Loehr, L.R.; Sotoodehnia, N.; Soliman, E.Z.; Alonso, A. American Heart Association's life simple 7 and risk of atrial fibrillation in a population without known cardiovascular disease: The ARIC (atherosclerosis risk in communities) study. *J. Am. Heart Assoc.* **2018**, *7*, e008424. [CrossRef] [PubMed]
6. Li, Y.; Pastori, D.; Guo, Y.; Wang, Y.; Lip, G.Y.H. Risk factors for new-onset atrial fibrillation: A focus on Asian populations. *Int. J. Cardiol.* **2018**, *261*, 92–98. [CrossRef] [PubMed]
7. Lloyd-Jones, D.M.; Hong, Y.; Labarthe, D.; Mozaffarian, D.; Appel, L.J.; Van Horn, L.; Greenlund, K.; Daniels, S.; Nichol, G.; Tomaselli, G.F.; et al. American Heart Association Strategic Planning Task Force and Statistics Committee Defining and setting national goals for cardiovascular health promotion and disease reduction: The American Heart Association's strategic impact goal through 2020 and beyond. *Circulation* **2010**, *121*, 586–613. [CrossRef] [PubMed]
8. Garg, P.K.; O'Neal, W.T.; Ogunsua, A.; Thacker, E.L.; Howard, G.; Soliman, E.Z.; Cushman, M. Usefulness of the American Heart Association's life simple 7 to predict the risk of atrial fibrillation (from the REasons for geographic and racial differences in stroke [REGARDS] study). *Am. J. Cardiol.* **2018**, *121*, 199–204. [CrossRef] [PubMed]
9. Isakadze, N.; Pratik, B.; Sandesara, B.; Patel, R.; Baer, J.; Isiadinso, I.; Alonso, A.; Lloyd, M.; Sperling, L. Life's simple 7 approach to atrial fibrillation prevention. *J. Atr. Fibrillation* **2018**, *11*, 2051. [CrossRef] [PubMed]
10. Pathak, R.K.; Middeldorp, M.E.; Lau, D.H.; Mehta, A.B.; Mahajan, R.; Twomey, D.; Alasady, M.; Hanley, L.; Antic, N.A.; McEvoy, R.D.; et al. Aggressive risk factor reduction study for atrial fibrillation and implications for the outcome of ablation: The ARREST-AF cohort study. *J. Am. Coll. Cardiol.* **2014**, *64*, 2222–2231. [CrossRef] [PubMed]
11. Hamada, R.; Lee, J.S.; Mori, K.; Watanabe, E.; Muto, S. Influence of abdominal obesity and habitual behaviors on incident atrial fibrillation in Japanese. *J. Cardiol.* **2018**, *71*, 118–124. [CrossRef] [PubMed]
12. Fatemi, O.; Yuriditsky, E.; Tsioufis, C.; Tsachris, D.; Morgan, T.; Basile, J.; Bigger, T.; Cushman, W.; Goff, D.; Soliman, E.Z.; et al. Impact of intensive glycemic control on the incidence of atrial fibrillation and associated cardiovascular outcomes in patients with type 2 diabetes mellitus (from the action to control cardiovascular risk in diabetes study). *Am. J. Cardiol.* **2014**, *114*, 1217–1222. [CrossRef] [PubMed]
13. Alonso, A.; Bahnson, J.L.; Gaussoin, S.A.; Bertoni, A.G.; Johnson, K.C.; Lewis, C.E.; Vetter, M.; Mantzoros, C.S.; Jeffery, R.W.; Soliman, E.Z. Look AHEAD Research Group Effect of an intensive lifestyle intervention on atrial fibrillation risk in individuals with type 2 diabetes: The Look AHEAD randomized trial. *Am. Heart J.* **2015**, *170*, 770–777.e5. [CrossRef] [PubMed]
14. Akesson, A.; Larsson, S.C.; Discacciati, A.; Wolk, A. Low-risk diet and lifestyle habits in the primary prevention of myocardial infarction in men: A population-based prospective cohort study. *J. Am. Coll. Cardiol.* **2014**, *64*, 1299–1306. [CrossRef] [PubMed]
15. Chomistek, A.K.; Chiuve, S.E.; Eliassen, A.H.; Mukamal, K.J.; Willett, W.C.; Rimm, E.B. Healthy lifestyle in the primordial prevention of cardiovascular disease among young women. *J. Am. Coll. Cardiol.* **2015**, *65*, 43–51. [CrossRef] [PubMed]
16. Csengeri, D.; Sprünker, N.A.; Di Castelnuovo, A.; Niiranen, T.; Vishram-Nielsen, J.K.; Costanzo, S.; Söderberg, S.; Jensen, S.M.; Vartiainen, E.; Donati, M.B.; et al. Alcohol consumption, cardiac biomarkers, and risk of atrial fibrillation and adverse outcomes. *Eur. Heart J.* **2021**, *42*, 1170–1177. [CrossRef] [PubMed]
17. Tada, H.; Kawashiri, M.A.; Yasuda, K.; Yamagishi, M. Associations between questionnaires on lifestyle and atherosclerotic cardiovascular disease in a Japanese general population: A cross-sectional study. *PLoS ONE* **2018**, *13*, e0208135. [CrossRef] [PubMed]

nutrients

Article

Fructose plus High-Salt Diet in Early Life Results in Salt-Sensitive Cardiovascular Changes in Mature Male Sprague Dawley Rats

Peter E. Levanovich [1], Charles S. Chung [1], Dragana Komnenov [2] and Noreen F. Rossi [1,2,3,*]

[1] Department of Physiology, Wayne State University, Detroit, MI 48201, USA; fy7541@med.wayne.edu (P.E.L.); cchung@wayne.edu (C.S.C.)
[2] Department of Internal Medicine, Wayne State University, Detroit, MI 48201, USA; fv6083@wayne.edu
[3] John D. Dingell VA Medical Center, Detroit, MI 48201, USA
* Correspondence: nrossi@wayne.edu

Abstract: Fructose and salt intake remain high, particularly in adolescents and young adults. The present studies were designed to evaluate the impact of high fructose and/or salt during pre- and early adolescence on salt sensitivity, blood pressure, arterial compliance, and left ventricular (LV) function in maturity. Male 5-week-old Sprague Dawley rats were studied over three 3-week phases (Phases I, II, and III). Two reference groups received either 20% glucose + 0.4% NaCl (GCS-GCS) or 20% fructose + 4% NaCl (FHS-FHS) throughout this study. The two test groups ingested fructose + 0.4% NaCl (FCS) or FHS during Phase I, then GCS in Phase II, and were then challenged with 20% glucose + 4% NaCl (GHS) in Phase III: FCS-GHS and FHS-GHS, respectively. Compared with GCS-GCS, systolic and mean pressures were significantly higher at the end of Phase III in all groups fed fructose during Phase I. Aortic pulse wave velocity (PWV) was elevated at the end of Phase I in FHS-GHS and FHS-FHS (vs. GCS-GCS). At the end of Phase III, PWV and renal resistive index were higher in FHS-GHS and FHS-FHS vs. GCS-GCS. Diastolic, but not systolic, LV function was impaired in the FHS-GHS and FHS-FHS but not FCS-FHS rats. Consumption of 20% fructose by male rats during adolescence results in salt-sensitive hypertension in maturity. When ingested with a high-salt diet during this early plastic phase, dietary fructose also predisposes to vascular stiffening and LV diastolic dysfunction in later life.

Keywords: aortic stiffness; fructose; glucose; hypertension; left ventricular diastolic dysfunction; pulse wave velocity; renal resistive index

1. Introduction

The prevalence of hypertension has been increasing in recent decades in the United States both independently and concurrently with diabetes [1]. Elevated fructose consumption has been implicated in metabolic disorders and subsequent cardiovascular morbidity [2–4]. In pre-clinical models, high levels of fructose consumption—often exceeding 60% of daily caloric intake—elicit hypertension and cardiovascular dysfunction, and implicate insulin signaling as the pathogenic mechanism [4,5]. Ingestion of 20% fructose in drinking water together with high-salt chow, which is more representative of the diet ingested by the upper quintile in humans in the United States, results in sodium and fluid retention in rats, enhanced sympathetic activation, and inadequate suppression of plasma renin activity, leading to a hypertensive state prior to development of frank metabolic syndrome or diabetes mellitus [6,7].

Adolescence is marked by the continuous development and growth of physiologic systems. In early stages of life, various systems undergo substantial ontogenetic changes, some of which are susceptible to modulation by external stimuli. Several studies have demonstrated the effect of excess fructose consumption on cardiovascular systems in adults [8–10]. However, little is understood regarding the impact of fructose-rich diets during adolescence on cardiovascular parameters later in life [11–15]. The major consumers of fructose are adolescents and young adults, with sugar-sweetened beverages representing the main source. Fructose intake in adolescents accounts for nearly 20% of daily energy consumption [16,17].

Western diets use high-fructose corn syrup extensively as a sweetener but are also high in sodium content [3]. Since pre-clinical studies indicate that a diet high in both fructose and salt results in hypertension [5,6,10,11], aortic stiffness, and early diastolic dysfunction [12], the question arises whether ingestion of high fructose and salt during a critical period early in life predisposes to salt-sensitive hypertension and cardiovascular dysfunction in later life. This window of plasticity during adolescence has been well recognized in behavioral science [18,19]. Likewise, with cardiovascular development, rat models have shown that interventions during critical time periods of ontogeny may modulate susceptibility to hypertension later in life. Insights into post-gestational influences on arterial pressure have been garnered predominantly from studies using genetically hypertensive-strain rats such as Dahl salt-sensitive and spontaneously hypertensive rats to investigate the impact on disease progression [20]. For example, four-week treatment of young spontaneously hypertensive rats with angiotensin-converting enzyme inhibition attenuated development of elevated blood pressure in later life [21]. The converse has not been given much attention, namely, whether factors such as diet or environment during this critical developmental period may adversely alter cardiovascular parameters in maturity, even in a rat strain that is not genetically prone to hypertension.

One in five adolescents in the United States are now considered pre-diabetic [22]. This increasing incidence of pre-diabetes raises the potential of cardiovascular dysfunction later in life that can be further impacted by poor dietary habits at this stage. Thus, the purpose of the present study was to investigate whether exposure to high fructose with or without high salt during the critical adolescent period will lead to hypertension and cardiovascular dysfunction in response to high-salt diet later in life. We hypothesized that rats consuming 20% fructose plus with 4% sodium diet during five to eight weeks of age (comparable to human pre- and early adolescence) [19,23] will develop elevated salt-sensitive blood pressure, reduced arterial compliance, and left ventricular diastolic dysfunction in adulthood when challenged with high dietary sodium in the absence of fructose.

2. Materials and Methods

All animal procedures and protocols were approved by the Wayne State University Institutional Animal Care and Use Committee (Protocol #19-03-1001). Animal care and experimentation was conducted in accordance with the guidelines and principles articulated in the National Institutes of Health Guide for the Care and Use of Laboratory Animals. Male Sprague Dawley rats (Envigo Sprague Dawley, Shelby, MI, USA) were housed under controlled conditions (21–23 °C; 12 h light and 12 h dark cycles, lighting period beginning at 6 a.m.).

2.1. Dietary Regimen

Upon arrival, rats were permitted to acclimate for at least 48 h and provided standard lab chow and water, ad libitum. As depicted in Figure 1, when rats reached ~4.5 weeks of age, a hemodynamic transmitter was implanted (as described in surgical procedures) and the animal was permitted to recover in individual standard polyurethane caging. One week later, rats were placed into metabolic housing units (Tecniplast USA, West Chester, PA, USA) and provided milled chow containing either 20% glucose and 0.4% Na$^+$ (glucose control salt, GCS; ModTest Diet® 5755-5WZZ; St. Louis, MO, USA) or 20% fructose and 0.4% Na$^+$ (fructose control salt, FCS; ModTest Diet® 5755-5W3Y; St. Louis, MO, USA). Rats were permitted a 3 day acclimation period followed by a 3 day baseline period where food and water were provided ad libitum and baseline hemodynamic data were recorded by telemetry. Then, the rats entered Phase I (Figure 1; study weeks 2 to 4, inclusive): GCS rats

(n = 9) continued on the same diet. Rats receiving FCS chow were then randomly assigned to continue FCS (n = 9) or placed on 20% fructose and 4.0% Na$^+$ (fructose high salt, FHS; ModTest Diet® 5755-5WZ8; n = 18; St. Louis, MO, USA) for three weeks. At this time, a pair feeding paradigm was initiated to achieve equal caloric intake among the groups on a day-to-day basis. Water continued to be provided ad libitum. Food and water intake and urine output were assessed daily. In Phase II (Figure 1, study weeks 5 to 7, inclusive), all rats were returned to standard individual shoebox housing units. Rats on GCS feed were maintained on this diet for the remainder of this study, including Phase III. Rats on FCS feed were then placed on GCS chow. The rats on FHS chow were then further randomly assigned to receive either GCS feed (n = 9) or to continue the FHS diet (n = 9). The rats on FHS chow during Phase II remained on FHS through to the end of this study.

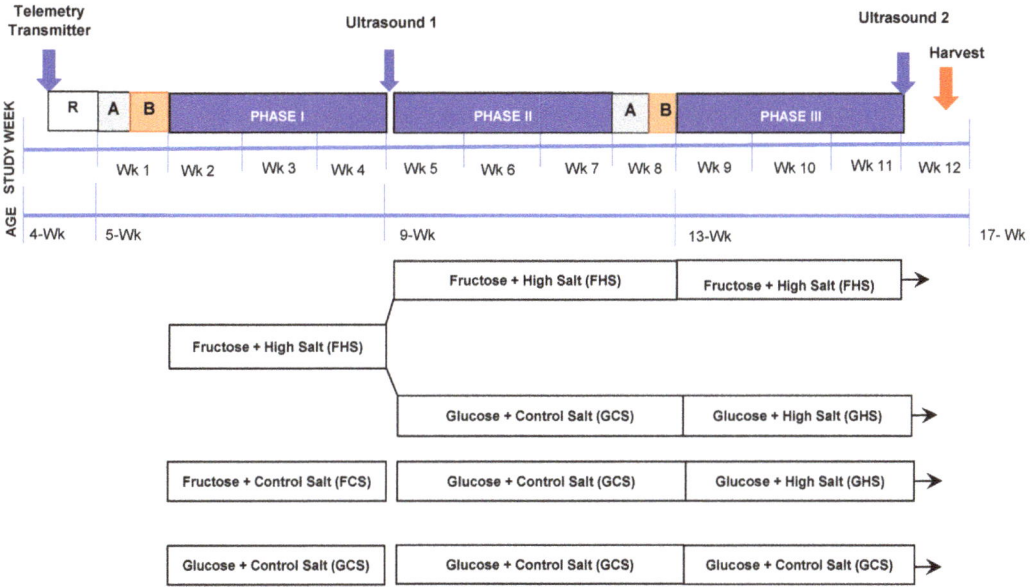

Figure 1. Schematic of the Timeline of Experimental Protocols and Study Phases. Rat age and study week are depicted across the timeline. R, recovery period; A, acclimation to metabolic cages; B, baseline. Surgery for telemetry transmitter placement and ultrasound studies are as indicated. Groups are subsequently depicted by their sugar-salt intake in Phases I and III.

After 3 weeks, the rats were again placed into metabolic cages and permitted to acclimate to the change in caging for three days prior to initiating Phase III (Figure 1; study weeks 9 to 11, inclusive). FCS- and FHS-fed rats that had been shifted to a GCS feed in Phase II were then subjected to a high-salt challenge without fructose for the remainder of the protocol using a 20% glucose and 4.0% Na$^+$ chow (glucose high salt, GHS; ModTest Diet® 5755-5WOW). This produced four groups characterized by their dietary regimens in the early and late phases—Phase 1 and Phase III, respectively (Figure 1). The groups are named based on their diets during Phases I and III: (a) GCS-GCS, (b) FCS-GHS, (c) FHS-GHS, and (d) FHS-FHS. Rats were maintained on these diets for an additional three weeks; thereafter, terminal studies were performed.

2.2. Ultrasonography

At the end of Phases I and III, rats were anesthetized in an induction chamber using 3% isoflurane and transferred to a pre-heated electronic ECG platform where 1–1.5% isoflurane was delivered via nosecone to maintain a sufficient plane of anesthesia. Fur from the chest and abdominal area was removed using an electric shaver followed by application of depilatory cream (Church & Dwight Co., Inc., Erwing, NJ, USA). Electrode gel was placed on each of the ECG strips where the rat's limbs were held in place using tape. Body temperature was measured via a rectal probe and contact gel preheated to 37 °C was applied before performing echocardiography according to standard methods [24,25].

Image acquisition was conducted using the Vevo3100 Imaging system and MX250S transducer (Fujifilm Visualsonics, Inc., Toronto, ON, Canada). Assessment of left ventricular (LV) dimensions and systolic function was performed using a short axis view in M-mode at the level of the papillary muscle. Left ventricular (LV) diastolic filling and function were assessed using pulsed wave Doppler of transmitral blood flow velocities. These were located using color imaging superimposed over an apical four-chamber view. Further assessment of LV diastolic function was conducted using tissue Doppler imaging (TDI) near the mitral annulus measured along the apical axis. Pulse wave velocity (PWV) determination within the aortic arch was made via the determination of pulse transit time from the aortic root to a point within the aortic arch. Distance between these points was measured using a B-mode image of this anatomical segment. Aortic PWV was calculated as the difference in pulse transit time (calculated using the ECG tracing as a reference) measured at these two points divided by the distance between them.

Renal resistive index (RRI) was determined using pulsed Doppler measurements along the left main renal artery. RRI was calculated by taking the difference between systolic and diastolic velocity divided by the diastolic velocity during each respective cardiac cycle [26]. Data analysis was performed offline using VevoLab and VevoVasc software (Fujifilm Visualsonics, Inc., Toronto, ON, Cananda) in blinded fashion.

2.3. Surgical Procedures

All surgical procedures were conducted under intraperitoneal ketamine (80 mg/kg; Mylan Institutional, LLC Rockford, IL, USA) and xylazine (10 mg/kg; Akorn Animal Health, Inc., Lake Forest, IL, USA) anesthesia and subcutaneous administration of buprenorphine SR (0.3 mg/kg) for analgesia.

Hemodynamic Transmitter Placement: Following right femoral artery isolation, a small arterial incision was made and the gel-filled catheter of the hemodynamic transmitter (HDS-10, Data Sciences International, New Brighton, MN, USA) was inserted into the vessel and advanced into the abdominal aorta. The catheter was then anchored in place to the femoral artery using 3-0 silk suture (Ethicon, Johnson & Johnson, New Brunswick, NJ, USA) and the transmitter body was subcutaneously tunneled to the right flank. Subcutaneous adipose tissue was reapproximated around the surgical sight and the incision was closed using surgical staples.

Vascular Catheter Placement: At the end of Phase III and after the second ultrasonography study, catheters were placed into the left carotid artery and external jugular vein using ketamine and xylazine as above, and previously performed in our laboratory [7,27]. Catheters were secured with 3-0 silk suture and tunneled subcutaneously to the base of the neck and exteriorized. All incisions were closed using 4-0 prolene suture (Ethicon, Johnson & Johnson, New Brunswick, NJ, USA). The catheters were then filled with heparinized saline (1000 units/mL). The rats were then permitted to recover in individually housed polyurethane cages.

2.4. Analytical Measurements and Calculations

Hemodynamic Telemetry: Acquisition of hemodynamic data was conducted using Ponemah software (Data Sciences International, New Brighton, MN, USA). Systolic blood pressure (SBP), diastolic blood pressure (DBP), mean arterial pressure (MAP), and heart rate (HR) were sampled for 10 s every 4 min at a sampling rate of 500 samples/second. Pulse pressure (PP) was calculated separately using these values. Baseline measurements were averaged over three days after cage acclimation. Sampling was performed at this rate continuously throughout Phases I and III within the metabolic cages.

Metabolic and Hormonal Assessment: During Phases I and III, daily chow consumption was measured gravimetrically and caloric and sodium (Na^+) intake values were determined based on dietary profiles for each feed.

At the end of Phase III and prior to terminal harvest, food was removed from caging at the beginning of the morning light cycles and terminal procedures were conducted at a minimum of 6 h later to promote a semi-fasting state (as permitted by our Animal Use Committee). Glucose levels were determined using a One-Touch Ultra glucose monitor (LifeScan, Inc., Malpitas, CA, USA) on 50 µL blood from the arterial catheter. Arterial blood was collected into pre-chilled tubes containing sodium ethylenediaminetetraacetic acid (EDTA) for plasma renin activity (PRA) and into separate pre-chilled tubes containing 120 µL of 500 mM sodium EDTA, 125 mM phenanthroline, 1 mM phenylmethanesulfonyl fluoride, 20 mM pepstatin, 1 mM enalapril and 10× phosphatase inhibitor cocktail for insulin determinations. Once collected, blood was immediately centrifuged at 3000 rpm for 4 min at 4 °C. Plasma was stored at −70 °C until assay. PRA and insulin levels were measured using a standard Elisa kits (IBL International, Hamburg, Germany and Bertin Pharma SAS, Montingny-le-Bretonneux, France, respectively) Insulin sensitivity was calculated using the ratio of plasma glucose to insulin levels.

Rats were euthanized using sodium pentobarbital (120 mg/kg, IV) and hearts were excised and preserved in formalin solution for 24–48 h before embedding for histological assessment. Samples were stained with Mason's Trichrome dye and images were acquired at 40× magnification (Leica CTR5000, Leica Microsystems Inc., Buffalo Grove, IL, USA).

Statistics: All values are presented as mean ± standard error (SE). One-way analysis of variance (ANOVA) was used to determine differences among groups with a Sidak's multiple comparisons test for post hoc analysis. Two-way ANOVAs with repeated measures were performed to compare differences over time using a Sidak's multiple comparisons test for post hoc analysis. A p-value less than 0.05 was considered statistically significant. Due to the technical nature of many of these experimental techniques and acquisition of data over an extended period, some data were not able to be acquired at each time point for each animal. When n-values deviate from the original assignment, the reason for missingness is provided and values imputed as the mean. Consistent with the use of a repeated measures design, animals with missing data in any phase were omitted from two-way ANOVA tests for the analysis of change over time.

3. Results
3.1. Metabolic and Humoral Profiles

Metabolic parameters are shown in Table 1. Initial and final rat weights did not differ among the groups on different dietary regimens. Plasma glucose and insulin levels did not vary among the groups and were comparable to either vendor specifications for standard Sprague Dawley rats on standard diets and rats fed control diets with no added sugar in similar studies [28–30]. The glucose:insulin ratio was significantly lower in the FHS-GHS and FHS-FHS groups.

Compared with the FCS-GHS group. Although the glucose:insulin ratio was nearly two-fold higher in the GCS-GCS rats compared with FHS-GHS and FHS-FHS rats, statistical significance was achieved only for the FHS-GHS ($p < 0.01$) but not for FHS-FHS groups ($p = 0.0512$). PRA was significantly reduced in FCS-GHS groups following high-salt challenge at the end of Phase III. FHS-GHS and FHS-FHS rats displayed a blunted inhibition of renin secretion.

Statistical differences among caloric intakes were observed following dietary changes from control salt to high-salt chow in Phase I, week 1 and in Phase III weeks 1 and 2 Caloric intakes were no different among the groups by of week 2 of Phase I and III except of the FCS-GHS group in Phase III that continued to ingest fewer calories (Table 2). Despite rigorous efforts to match intake among the groups, rats in the FHS-GHS and FHS-FHS diets had lower caloric intake only in week 1 of Phase I (and consequently lower calorie and sodium intakes compared with weeks 2 and 3 of Phase I, $p < 0.05$ vs. either calorie or sodium, respectively) after which their caloric intake was no different than that of the GCS-GCS group. High salt-fed rats consumed approximately 10-fold greater amount of sodium than that consumed by the control salt-fed rats, consistent with their respective dietary sodium diets.

Table 1. Initial and Final Body Weights, Heart Weights, Glycemic Parameters and Plasma Renin Activity among the Four Groups of Rats.

Dietary Regimen	n	Initial Weight (g)	Final Weight (g)	Heart Weight (g/kg)	Fasting Glucose (mg/dL)	Fasting Insulin (ng/mL)	G:I Ratio ($\times 10^6$)	PRA (ngAngI/mL/hr)
GCS-GCS	9	125 ± 4	381 ± 9	3.3 ± 0.1	128 ± 13	1.14 ± 0.23	64.7 ± 6.4	1.82 ± 0.20
FCS-GHS	9	132 ± 4	347 ± 10	3.4 ± 0.1	129 ± 24	0.74 ± 0.12	74.6 ± 12.6	0.66 ± 0.12 *
FHS-GHS	8	128 ± 3	362 ± 12	3.2 ± 0.1	126 ± 14	1.33 ± 0.12	31.6 ± 1.9 *,†	1.35 ± 0.28
FHS-FHS	9	127 ± 5	366 ± 12	3.4 ± 0.1	118 ± 11	1.03 ± 0.17	39.1 ± 7.1 †	1.09 ± 0.29

GCS-GCS, 20% glucose + 0.4% NaCl in Phases I–III; FCS-GHS, 20% fructose + 0.4% NaCl in Phase 1 and 20% glucose +4% NaCl in Phase III; FHS-GHS, 20% fructose + 4% NaCl in Phase 1 and 20% glucose + 4% NaCl in Phase III; FHS-FHS, 20% fructose + 4% NaCl in Phases I–III. PRA, plasma renin activity; G:I Ratio, glucose:insulin ratio. All groups except FHS-FHS were on 20% glucose + 0.4% NaCl in Phase II. Due to lack of sufficient plasma for insulin, n values for insulin and G:I Ratio are as follows: 5, 6, 7 and 7. Values are the mean ± SE; n as indicated per group. * $p < 0.05$ vs. GCS-GCS. † $p < 0.05$ vs. FCS-GHS.

Table 2. Daily Caloric and Sodium Consumption.

		PHASE I					
		WEEK 1		WEEK 2		WEEK 3	
Dietary Regimen	n	Caloric Intake (kcal/day)	Sodium Intake (mmol/day)	Caloric Intake (kcal/day)	Sodium Intake (mmol/day)	Caloric Intake (kcal/day)	Sodium Intake (mmol/day)
GCS-GCS	9	61.5 ± 1.7	3.0 ± 0.3	68.4 ± 1.3	3.0 ± 0.1	66.0 ± 2.1	2.9 ± 0.1
FCS-GHS	9	60.7 ± 2.6	2.7 ± 0.1	67.2 ± 1.4	3.0 ± 0.1	65.7 ± 2.0	3.2 ± 0.3
FHS-GHS	8	48.7 ± 1.6 *,†	23.5 ± 0.8 *,†	60.6 ± 2.2 *	29.2 ± 1.1 *,†	61.8 ± 2.1	29.3 ± 0.9 *,†
FHS-FHS	9	51.9 ± 2.1 *,†	24.9 ± 1.0 *,†	63.9 ± 1.2	30.9 ± 0.6 *,†	63.5 ± 1.5	31.0 ± 0.8 *,†
		PHASE III					
		WEEK 1		WEEK 2		WEEK 3	
Dietary Regimen	n	Caloric Intake (kcal/day)	Sodium Intake (mmol/day)	Caloric Intake (kcal/day)	Sodium Intake (mmol/day)	Caloric Intake (kcal/day)	Sodium Intake (mmol/day)
GCS-GCS	9	62.6 ± 1.9	2.8 ± 0.1	63.5 ± 2.1	2.9 ± 0.1	64.3 ± 1.8	2.8 ± 0.1
FCS-GHS	9	45.9 ± 1.7 *	22.1 ± 0.8 *	54.4 ± 1.4 *	26.2 ± 0.7 *	57.1 ± 1.3	27.5 ± 0.6 *
FHS-GHS	8	50.1 ± 2.5 *	23.3 ± 1.2 *	56.1 ± 2.2	26.0 ± 0.8 *	59.9 ± 2.0	27.7 ± 0.6 *
FHS-FHS	9	60.5 ± 1.6 †,§	27.5 ± 0.8 *	63.9 ± 1.9 †,§	29.0 ± 0.3 *	66.4 ± 2.6 †	29.9 ± 1.0 *

Values are the mean ± SE, n as indicated per group. Group names as in Table 1. Caloric intake calculated using caloric profiles of 3.98 kcal/g and 3.61 kcal/g for 0.4% and 4% NaCl chow, respectively. * $p < 0.05$ vs. GCS-GCS; † $p < 0.05$ vs. FCS-GHS; § $p < 0.05$ vs. FHS-GHS.

3.2. Hemodynamic Effects

In Phase I, the addition of high salt in the diet of fructose-fed rats led to a progressive increase in mean arterial pressure that was significantly elevated after four days (data not shown). This increase was sustained for the subsequent two weeks. By the end of Phase I, the MAP increased in all groups consistent with expected changes in blood pressure with maturation; however, MAP was significantly higher in the rats receiving FHS diet during this phase (Table 3A). The FCS-GHS and FHS-GHS groups received GCS chow during Phase II and MAP at the beginning of Phase III did not differ from the MAP of the GCS-GCS group (data not shown). When FCS-GHS and FHS-GHS groups were placed on the GHS diet in Phase III, significant increases in MAP occurred within 1 week and these were sustained throughout the remainder of the phase. Final MAP pressure levels were comparable to those of FHS-FHS rats that had been on high-salt diet throughout all three phases (Table 3B). Systolic blood pressures at increased significantly in all groups on high-salt diet during Phase III compared with the GCS-GCS group that had ingested glucose and 0.4% salt chow throughout this study ($p < 0.05$). Diastolic blood pressures at the end of Phase I did not differ across any of the groups; therefore, the increases in MAP were driven predominately by systolic mechanisms. Pulse pressure, however, did not increase significantly. Additionally, no differences existed among groups when heart rate was assessed.

Table 3. Hemodynamic Parameters in the Four Groups of Rats at Baseline and End of Phase 1 and Phase 3.

		(A)			
Dietary Regimen		MAP (mmHg)		HEART RATE (BPM)	
	n	Baseline	End Phase I	Baseline	End Phase I
GCS-GCS	9	100.0 ± 1.0	108.4 ± 1.6	465 ± 8	391 ± 16
FCS-GHS	9	100.7 ± 0.9	108.0 ± 0.9	458 ± 9	395 ± 15
FHS-GHS	8	100.6 ± 1.3	111.1 ± 1.3	456 ± 11	381 ± 8
FHS-FHS	9	99.4 ± 1.0	110.2 ± 1.4	451 ± 11	391 ± 11
		(B)			
Dietary Regimen	n	Δ MAP (mmHg)	Δ SBP (mmHg)	Δ DBP (mmHg)	Δ HR (BPM)	Δ PP (MMHG)
GCS-GCS	7	10 ± 1.0	11 ± 2.2	11 ± 1.2	−92 ± 11	2.4 ± 1.5
FCS-GHS	8	15 ± 0.9 *	18 ± 0.9 *	14 ± 1.3	−103 ± 18	4.2 ± 1.6
FHS-GHS	8	15 ± 1.4 *	18 ± 1.7 *	13 ± 1.7	−105 ± 6	4.2 ± 2.0
FHS-FHS	8	16 ± 2.0 **	19 ± 2.3 **	14 ± 1.9	−89 ± 14	4.6 ± 1.4

Group names as in Table 1. Values are the mean ± SE, n as indicated per group. (**A**) Mean arterial pressure (MAP) and heart rate (HR) at baseline and at the end of Phase I. (**B**) Study-wide changes in hemodynamics calculated as the difference between measurements taken at the end of Phase III and baseline values at the beginning of Phase I. Values are the mean ± SE, n as indicated per group. * $p < 0.05$ vs. GCS-GCS; ** $p < 0.01$ vs. GCS-GCS.

3.3. Measurements of Vascular Compliance

Echocardiography and ultrasonography studies were performed upon completion of Phases I and III. At the end of Phase I, FHS diet significantly increased PWV of the ascending thoracic aorta, thereby indicating decreased aortic compliance compared to the GCS-GCS group (Figure 2). By the end of Phase III, maintenance of the FHS diet throughout all three phases of the protocol led to a significantly greater PWV in the in FHS-FHS group compared with the GCS-GCS group that had glucose and control salt diet for the same duration. Notably, PWV was significantly higher in the FHS-FHS group at the end of Phase III compared with the same animals at the end of Phase I.

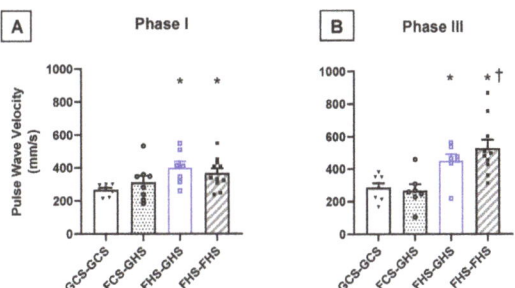

Figure 2. Pulse Wave Velocity at the end of Phases I and III. Pulse wave velocity (PWV) of the ascending aorta assessed (**A**) at the end of Phase I and (**B**) at the end of Phase III. Group labels are as described in the legend for Table 1. Values are the mean ± SE; n as depicted on the graphs. * $p < 0.05$ vs. GCS-GCS (by one-way ANOVA); † $p < 0.05$ vs. FHS-FHS in Phase I (by two-way ANOVA with repeated measures).

No differences were observed in the RRI among any of the groups at the end of Phase I (Figure 3). Similar to PWV values, FHS-GHS and FHS-FHS groups in Phase III displayed a statistically higher RRI than GCS-GCS rats. These trends were only elevated in Phase III and demonstrated no intra-group variability when compared to Phase I by two-way ANOVA. Note that due to anatomic and/or technical reasons, PWV and RRI were not able to be reliably assessed in each animal.

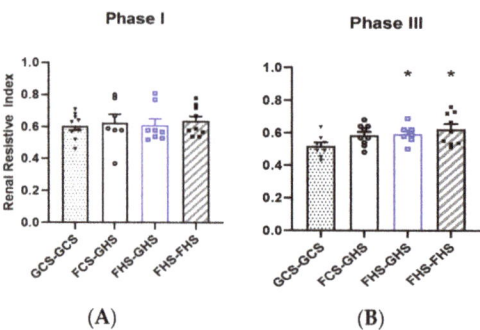

Figure 3. Renal Resistive Index at the end of Phases I and III. Renal resistive index (RRI) of the left main renal artery using doppler imaging (**A**) at the end of Phase I and (**B**) at the end of Phase III. Values are the mean ± SE; *n* as depicted on the graphs. * $p < 0.05$ vs. GCS-GCS in Phase III.

3.4. Echocardiographic Assessments

Physical assessment of the LV was performed using a short axis view and M-mode imaging. Table 4 depicts the results of echocardiography of the LV performed at the end of Phase III. No significant differences of standard systolic function, such as ejection fraction and fractional shortening, were observed among the groups. LV mass was significantly greater in the FHS-GHS and FHS-FHS groups vs. the GCS-GCS group. Further assessment of structural morphology revealed significant increases in anterior and posterior wall thickness in the FHS-GHS group. These changes were only apparent during diastole. In the FHS-FHS group, LV thickness only reached significance in the anterior wall. When assessed as a ratio of total wall thickness (sum of anterior and posterior walls) to inner diameter of the LV during diastole, there was a significant reduction in the ratio in FHS-GHS rats when compared with that of the GCS-GCS group (Figure 4A–D). Figure 4E shows histological views typical of the LV myocardium from the four groups. Notably, collagen staining was observed in the tissues taken from the FHS-GHS and FHS-FHS rats. Taken together, these measurements are consistent with ventricular hypertrophy and concentric remodeling.

Figure 5A shows representative Doppler images of transmitral flow from GCS-GCS and FHS-FHS rats at the end of Phase III. Table 5 shows values of diastolic function conducted by way of pulsed and tissue Doppler imaging at the end of Phase III. The ratio of early to late phase filling (E/A) demonstrated a significant reduction in the FHS-FHS group compared with the GCS-GCS group. The E/A ratios for each of the groups at the end of both Phase I and Phase III indicate that this parameter of diastolic dysfunction is significantly suppressed only after 12 weeks of the diet high in both fructose and salt (Figure 5B). Reductions in the E/A ratio in the FCS-GHS and FHS-GHS test groups were also observed, although these values did not achieve significance ($p = 0.064$ vs. GCS-GCS). Likewise, decreases in mitral valve deceleration time were also observed across all groups when compared to the GCS-GCS group. However, these were also only significant in the FHS-FHS group.

Table 4. Echocardiographic Parameters at the End of Phase III.

	Groups			
	GCS-GCS	FCS-GHS	FHS-GHS	FHS-FHS
n	9	8	8	9
LVEF (%)	74.9 ± 3.4	77.3 ± 4.4	80.3 ± 3.7	78.2 ± 2.3
LVFS (%)	46.0 ± 3.4	49.1 ± 4.4	51.9 ± 4.4	48.8 ± 2.4
$LVID_S$ (mm)	3.7 ± 0.3	3.4 ± 0.4	3.0 ± 0.4	3.5 ± 0.3
$LVID_D$ (mm)	6.7 ± 0.3	6.5 ± 0.3	6.1 ± 0.4	6.9 ± 0.4
$LVAW_S$ (mm)	3.2 ± 0.1	3.3 ± 0.2	3.5 ± 0.2	3.6 ± 0.1
$LVAW_D$ (mm)	1.9 ± 0.03	2.0 ± 0.1	2.5 ± 0.1 *	2.2 ± 0.1 *
$LVPW_S$ (mm)	3.5 ± 0.1	3.5 ± 0.2	4.0 ± 0.3	4.0 ± 0.2
$LVPW_D$ (mm)	2.3 ± 0.1	2.4 ± 0.1	3.0 ± 0.3 *	2.7 ± 0.2
$LVTW_S$ (mm)	6.8 ± 0.2	6.8 ± 0.4	7.4 ± 0.3	7.6 ± 0.4
$LVTW_D$ (mm)	4.3 ± 0.1	4.4 ± 0.2	5.6 ± 0.4 *	4.9 ± 0.3
LV Mass (mg)	1190 ± 73	1060 ± 59	1401 ± 56 *	1373.0 ± 75 *

Group names as in Table 1: LVEF, left ventricular ejection fraction; LVFS, left ventricular fractional shortening; $LVID_S$, left ventricular systolic internal diameter; $LVID_D$, left ventricular diastolic internal diameter; LVAW, left ventricular anterior wall width; LVPW, left ventricular posterior wall width; LVTW, left ventricular total wall width; LV Mass, left ventricular mass. Values are the mean ± SE. * $p < 0.05$ vs. GCS-GCS.

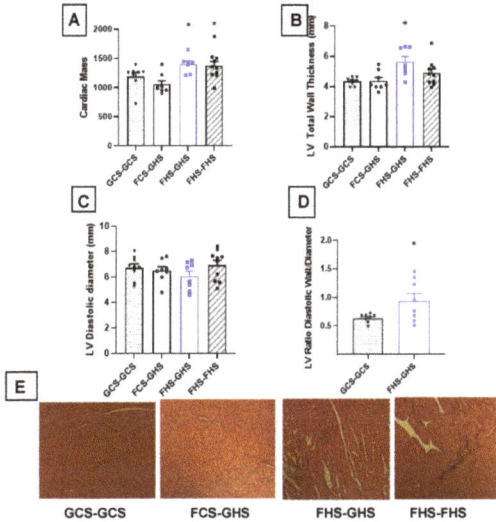

Figure 4. Assessment of Left Ventricular Parameters in Phase III. Images were acquired using a short axis view of the left ventricle (LV) via M-Mode. (**A**) Cardiac mass was the total wet weight of the heart after harvesting. (**B**) Total wall thickness was the sum of anterior and posterior LV wall widths. (**C**) LV diastolic diameter was the diameter of the LV at end diastole. (**D**) LV diastolic wall/diameter was calculated as the ratio of total wall thickness to the diameter of the LV at end-diastole. Values are the mean ± SE, n as indicated per group; * $p < 0.05$ vs. GCS-GCS. (**E**) Representative histological sections of LV tissue from each group. Group labels are as described in the legend for Table 1. Mason's trichrome; 40× magnification.

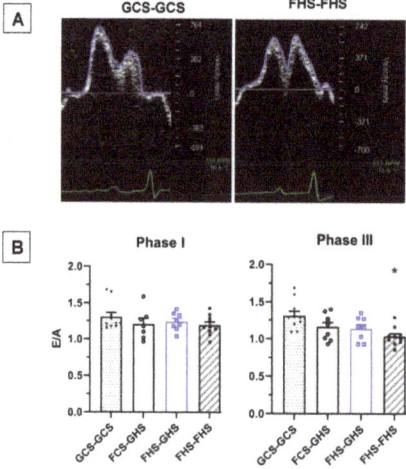

Figure 5. Assessment of Diastolic Function. (**A**) Representative Doppler images of transmitral flow patterns from GCS-GCS and FHS-FHS rats at the end of Phase III. (**B**) Ratio of early (E-wave) to late (A-wave) left ventricular filling (E-wave) left ventricular filling as index of diastolic function. Group labels are as described in the legend for Table 1. Values are the mean ± SE; n as indicated per group, * $p < 0.05$ vs. GCS-GCS.

Table 5. Echocardiographic Parameters Associated with Diastolic Function at the End of Phase III.

	Group			
	GCS-GCS	FCS-GHS	FHS-GHS	FHS-FHS
n	9	8	8	9
Peak E (mm/s)	706 ± 22	630 ± 45	652 ± 41	641 ± 39
Peak A (mm/s)	555 ± 27	550 ± 44	576 ± 34	621 ± 32
E/A	1.31 ± 0.06	1.16 ± 0.06	1.14 ± 0.06	1.03 ± 0.04 **
DT (ms)	39.5 ± 4.0	28.0 ± 2.2 *	31.8 ± 3.0	25.4 ± 2.3 **
IVRT (ms)	25.5 ± 1.0	27.7 ± 1.5	27.6 ± 1.1	29.0 ± 0.9
E' (mm/s)	34.1 ± 2.6	32.3 ± 4.6	34.2 ± 4.0	27.4 ± 1.8
A' (mm/s)	45.3 ± 3.7	45.8 ± 4.7	48.0 ± 4.9	47.1 ± 4.7
E/E'	22.5 ± 1.9	25.2 ± 6.2	21.1 ± 3.3	24.3 ± 2.3
E'/A'	0.81 ± 0.01	0.71 ± 0.09	0.81 ± 0.15	0.64 ± 0.01

Group names as in Table 1: E, early phase ventricular filling; A, late phase ventricular filling; DT, mitral valve deceleration time; IVRT, isovolumetric relaxation time; E', mitral annulus early phase filling; A', mitral annulus late phase filling. Values are the mean ± SE. * $p < 0.05$ vs. GCS-GCS, ** $p < 0.01$ vs. GCS-GCS.

4. Discussion

The major findings of this study support the hypothesis that consumption of fructose plus high-salt diet during pre- and early adolescence results in measurable deleterious cardiovascular effects in adulthood when ingesting high dietary sodium without fructose. Specifically, ingestion of high fructose either alone or with high salt during this early critical period of life resulted in salt-sensitive hypertension in maturity, despite the rats resuming a diet that was free of fructose and had normal salt content during young adulthood. The elevation in mean and systolic blood pressures in FCS-GHS and FHS-GHS rats was comparable to rats that had ingested high-fructose and high-salt diet throughout the entire protocol. The cardiovascular parameters such as aortic and renal artery compliance, LV mass and wall thickness, and LV diastolic function were impaired only in the rats that had ingested high fructose and high salt during adolescence. Notably, the magnitude of salt-sensitive blood pressure elevation was similar in all groups fed fructose in early life. Taken together, these findings suggest that the reduced vascular compliance and LV diastolic dysfunction are not simply due to the elevated blood pressure or fructose alone in early life but to the combination of fructose with high salt in adolescence.

An extensive body of work has accrued to show that maternal exposure to environmental and dietary conditions can profoundly influence not only fetal development but also subsequent cardiac and renal function in offspring [31]. Importantly, moderately high maternal salt with [32] or without [33,34] concurrent fructose intake leads to hypertension in male rats. In contrast, the impact of factors on cardiovascular function in the adolescent period of plasticity has received scant attention.

The comparable increases in MAP in each of the four groups during Phase I was consistent with the ~10 mmHg increase typically observed as rats grow and mature [35]. Except for the FHS-FHS group that entered Phase III with elevated blood pressure, rats in the other groups, all of which were on GCS during Phase II, entered Phase III with normal MAPs similar to the GCS-GCS control group. The hypertension that developed in response to high-salt intake in rats that ingested fructose during the critical developmental period was driven by elevation in systolic pressure to levels equivalent to the rats that had consumed fructose and high salt throughout. Slight increases in diastolic blood pressure occurred which prevented any statistically significant increases in pulse pressure which were, nonetheless, nearly two-fold higher than in the GCS-GCS group. Importantly, systolic blood pressure and pulse pressure are strongly correlated with subsequent major adverse cardiac events [36,37]. Thus, fructose alone or combined with high salt during the critical adolescent period predisposes to salt sensitivity and hypertension in maturity.

The mechanisms underlying later salt-sensitive hypertension in rats that consumed fructose in youth remain to be defined. Failure to suppress PRA in the FHS-GHS and FHS-FHS suggests involvement of the renin-angiotensin system. Angiotensin II serves as a pressor inducing hormone that can act systemically on the vasculature to increase vasoconstriction or on target organs such as the kidney to increase extracellular fluid volume by facilitating fluid reabsorption [38]. Notably, adult rats fed similar fructose and high-salt diets exhibit increased proximal tubular sodium-hydrogen exchange [39–42] and stimulation of thick ascending limb sodium-potassium-2-chloride cotransporter expression [43] as well as enhanced renal sympathetic nerve activity [7]. Increased extracellular volume due to positive net sodium balance together with neurohumorally mediated vasoconstriction over the course of Phase III in rats fed a high-fructose diet in Phase I likely plays a role in producing the increases in MAP [6]. However, increased extracellular volume is unlikely to be the only governing factor. Prolonged fructose feeding has been associated with hyperinsulinemia which can cause increased levels of other vasoactive factors such as endothelin-1 [28], reactive oxygen species and uric acid [4,27,44–47]. Although no differences in basal plasma glucose or insulin levels were observed among all four groups, the significantly lower glucose:insulin ratio in the groups that consumed fructose and high salt in adolescence indicates a possible role for insulin resistance, a hallmark of pre-diabetes. Whether these or other mechanisms remain "primed" by high-fructose intake during the plastic adolescent period and are then brought into play to induce hypertension upon ingestion of high-salt diet in the absence of fructose later in life will need further investigation.

Increased arterial pressure over time can induce cellular and molecular alterations that deform the vascular wall and increase afterload to the left ventricle [48]. It is noteworthy that the FCS-GHS group displayed hypertension equivalent to that of the other fructose-fed groups by the end of Phase III, but vascular stiffening and LV diastolic dysfunction occurred only in the groups exposed to both fructose and high salt in early life. In fact, evidence of vascular dysfunction became evident in FHS groups by the end of Phase I as demonstrated by increased PWV despite similar arterial pressures across all groups. In Phase III, PWV is augmented in both FHS-GCS and FHS-FHS groups when compared to Phase III GCS-GCS controls. Notably, in rats fed fructose and high salt for the entire protocol, the decline in aortic compliance progressed further in Phase III when compared to initial Phase I measurements. These findings suggest that the combination of fructose and high-salt diet has a direct effect on vascular function that is independent of the elevated arterial pressure. Failure of optimal suppression of PRA in the FHS-GHS and FHS-FHS groups supports an angiotensin-associated mechanism underlying the reduced arterial compliance in these groups, but does not exclude additional potential mechanisms such as increased sympathetic activity [7] or increased sodium reabsorption that could lead to an expanded extracellular volume [39–41]. Notably, these mechanisms are not necessarily independent of each other as increased renal sympathetic activity enhances renin secretion and Ang II increases proximal tubule sodium reabsorption by the kidney. Importantly, the present data indicate that fructose alone during the early adolescent phase does not impair the normal suppression of PRA with ingestion of high salt later in life. Rather the combined ingestion of fructose and high salt in this early plastic phase does predispose to salt-sensitive hypertension later in life.

Several studies have demonstrated the prognostic ability of the renal resistive index (RRI) to predict the decline in renal function associated with the progression of hypertension, chronic nephropathy, and diabetes mellitus in humans [49–52] and adverse cardiac and renal outcomes in hypertension [53,54]. While some controversy remains over the reliability of RRI as a measurement across all diseases [55], there is a general consensus that elevated RRI is linked closely with systemic vascular stiffness. Additional studies have found functional correlation between elevated RRI and intrarenal perfusion as well as histopathological findings such as tubulointerstitial damage and renal atherosclerosis [56–58].

Consistent with PWV, we observed significant increases in RRI in each of the groups fed fructose in early adolescence only in Phase III. Importantly, as a measure of pulsatility, RRI reflects intrinsic renal artery compliance but is also influenced substantially by changes in upstream systemic and downstream intrarenal vascular properties [26]. The elevated RRI is thus consistent with the increased aortic PWV observed in this present study but suggests that the decline in renal artery compliance is delayed compared with changes in the ascending aorta and aortic arch where hydrostatic and shear forces are greater [59]. Oxidative stress [27,47], impaired nitric oxide generation [6], and inflammatory mechanisms [60] have been implicated in vascular changes during fructose and high-salt exposure. Again, whether these same factors contribute to the impaired compliance of the aorta and renal artery observed after exposure to fructose and high salt in youth is likely but remains to be proven.

Total peripheral resistance is a function of MAP and heart rate—an increase in either factor without a corresponding decrease in the other elevates total peripheral resistance [61]. In the present study, this physiologic dysfunction was observed as both an increase in systemic resistance and lack of vascular compliance. The net effect of these factors was an increase in ventricular afterload leading to left ventricular remodeling and subsequent hypertrophy evidenced by increased LV mass and total wall thickness. Together with the augmented ratio of ventricular wall thickness to end-diastolic cavity radius, these findings are consistent with concentric remodeling with preserved ejection fraction [62,63]. The decrease in the ratio of early to late diastolic filling was accompanied by an increase in isovolumetric relaxation time and decrease in mitral valve deceleration time. Shortening of the mitral valve deceleration time implies restrictive filling and has been positively correlated to severe adverse cardiac events [64]. Each of these measurements are indicative of diastolic dysfunction and are phenotypes associated with either the development of cardiomyopathy in rats that had consumed fructose and high salt in the critical adolescent period [65–68]. Despite the lack of rigorous morphometric studies, collagen deposition was apparent only in the two groups of rats fed FHS in early life. The present finding is consistent with the findings of Abdelhaffez et al. [69] who reported increased cardiac interstitial fibrosis after rats ingested 12 weeks of 20% fructose in their drinking water. Unfortunately, that study did not provide functional data. Intriguingly, long-chain non-coding mRNAs that are co-expressed with mRNAs involved the fructose metabolic pathways have been implicated in myocardial fibrosis after myocardial infarction in humans [70]. Whether similar cellular and biochemical pathways are implicated in fructose-high salt-induced cardiovascular dysfunction will be crucial avenues of investigation.

4.1. Limitations

The present study used 20% glucose with 0.4% NaCl as the reference group to control for caloric intake rather than a standard rat chow which is typically ~7% simple sugars. Previous studies have found no significant changes in arterial pressure or bodily sodium balance in rats fed 20% glucose with either low- or high-salt diet for short (1 week) or more prolonged periods of time (3 weeks) [6,7]. It should be noted that in these other studies, the sugars (glucose and fructose) were in the drinking water rather than in the chow. Incorporating the carbohydrate in the chow permitted more accurate assessment of intake and equalization across groups. Nonetheless, it is important to note that, while the timeline of the study at present exceeds that of these prior studies, the values for hemodynamic, vascular, and cardiac parameters are comparable in our GCS-GCS rats that we used as reference group to parameters observed after three weeks of 20% glucose in drinking water with either 0.4% or 4% NaCl [27]. The 9- to 10-week exposure to dietary fructose in the FHS-FHS group was certainly longer than that in previous studies that evaluated these cardiovascular parameters. PRA was not suppressed in the FCS-FHS and the FHS-FHS groups. Ideally, concurrent plasma Ang II measurements would have been confirmatory as in our previous studies [7,27]. The volume of plasma required for plasma Ang II measurements by validated assay in our laboratory is 0.8–1.0 mL. Obtaining blood from conscious rats via indwelling catheter while avoiding hypotension that could potentially induce an increase in PRA and Ang II independent of the dietary condition was a primary goal. Due to the need to assess other plasma factors, we were only able to obtain sufficient plasma to reliably assess PRA, which only required 50 µL of plasma. Sex hormones play an important role in the development of hypertension following a high-fructose diet [71,72]. We only studied male rats in the present cohort in part due to restrictions in the number of animals permitted during the pandemic restrictions. We acknowledge that female rats have been shown to be particularly resistant to the development of insulin resistance and, therefore, may prove to be less prone to the consequences of fructose and high-salt diet [73–75]. Studies in female rats will be needed in the future. Finally, the nature of the ultrasonographic imaging precluded obtaining all parameters in each of the rats due to anatomical variations or issues with technique. Blood samples obtained at the end of this study via the indwelling arterial catheter were performed in conscious animals to avoid confounders such as hypotension and anesthesia; however, in some cases, this limited the volume of plasma that could be obtained due clotting or kinking of the catheter. Although statistical analyses for missing data were performed by imputation using the mean, the limitation still exists.

4.2. Perspectives

Pre-clinical and clinical studies have clearly shown the relationship between frank diabetes mellitus and cardiovascular complications [65,76–80]. Insulin resistance in the pre-diabetic state even without frank hyperglycemia may play an important role in developing cardiovascular abnormalities [81]. Alternatively, the exposure to both fructose *and* high salt early in life in Phase I is an important factor for later development of the vasculopathy and cardiomyopathy.

On the other hand, fructose feeding alone, without the addition of high dietary sodium during the critical developmental period is sufficient to induce as state of salt sensitivity later in life which renders the body susceptible to hypertension. Chronically this can lead to various cardiac and renal co-morbidities such as heart failure and chronic kidney disease [82,83]. Even FCS-GHS groups that became hypertensive only later in life had a reduction in diastolic function, indicated by the E/A ratio, but this was not significant. Contrastingly, the addition of high salt to a moderate fructose diet during pubescent, developmental years had lasting effects on cardiac and renal function evidenced by diastolic dysfunction, ventricular hypertrophy, and failed renin suppression. This detriment occurred in rats that were fed this fructose and high-salt diet chronically and those that were allowed a period of reprise from poor dietary conditions (FHS-GHS) groups. Indeed, diets with fructose fed early in life-with or without the presence of elevated sodium—promote adaptations that render the body increasingly vulnerable to complications caused by even modest dietary insults; these insults are long lasting and with severe consequence.

5. Conclusions

In summary, consumption of 20% fructose but not glucose by male rats during pre- and early adolescence, a proportion of caloric intake comparable to the upper quintile of humans, results in salt-sensitive hypertension in mature animals. When ingested together with a high-salt diet during this critical plastic phase, dietary fructose also predisposes to vascular stiffening and left ventricular diastolic dysfunction in later life.

Author Contributions: Conceptualization, N.F.R. and P.E.L.; methodology, N.F.R., P.E.L. and C.S.C.; software, C.S.C., P.E.L. and N.F.R.; validation, N.F.R.; formal analysis, P.E.L., C.S.C. and N.F.R.; investigation, P.E.L., D.K. and N.F.R.; resources, N.F.R.; data curation, N.F.R.; writing—original draft preparation, P.E.L.; writing—review and editing, N.F.R., C.S.C. and D.K.; visualization, P.E.L. and N.F.R.; supervision, N.F.R.; project administration, N.F.R.; funding acquisition, N.F.R. All authors have read and agreed to the published version of the manuscript.

Funding: This work was funded by a Merit Grant from the Dept. of Veterans Affairs #RX000851 to NFR, R01HL151738 to CSC, and graduate fellowship by NIH 2T32HL120822 for PEL.

Institutional Review Board Statement: All animal procedures and protocols were conducted according to the guidelines of the Declaration of Helsinki approved by the Wayne State University Institutional Animal Care and Use Committee (Protocol #19-03-1001). Animal care and experimentation were further conducted in accordance with the guidelines and principles articulated in the National Institutes of Health Guide for the Care and Use of Laboratory Animals.

Informed Consent Statement: Not applicable.

Data Availability Statement: The data presented in this study are available on request from the corresponding author by formal request to the Research and Development Office of the John D. Dingell VA Medical Center, Detroit, Michigan.

Acknowledgments: The authors thank Min Wu for her technical assistance.

Conflicts of Interest: The authors declare no conflict of interest.

References

1. Ostchega, Y.; Fryar, C.D.; Nwankwo, T.; Nguyen, D.T. Hypertension Prevalence Among Adults Aged 18 and Over: United States, 2017–2018. NCHS Data Brief. 2020; pp. 1–8. Available online: https://www.cdc.gov/nchs/products/databriefs/db364.htm (accessed on 1 September 2021).
2. Bray, G.A.; Nielsen, S.J.; Popkin, B.M. Consumption of high-fructose corn syrup in beverages may play a role in the epidemic of obesity. *Am. J. Clin. Nutr.* **2004**, *79*, 537–543. [CrossRef]
3. Tappy, L.; Le, K.A. Metabolic effects of fructose and the worldwide increase in obesity. *Physiol. Rev.* **2010**, *90*, 23–46. [CrossRef] [PubMed]
4. Tran, L.T.; Yuen, V.G.; McNeill, J.H. The fructose-fed rat: A review on the mechanisms of fructose-induced insulin resistance and hypertension. *Mol. Cell Biochem.* **2009**, *332*, 145–159. [CrossRef]
5. Martinez, F.J.; Rizza, R.A.; Romero, J.C. High-fructose feeding elicits insulin resistance, hyperinsulinism, and hypertension in normal mongrel dogs. *Hypertension* **1994**, *23*, 456–463. [CrossRef]
6. Gordish, K.L.; Kassem, K.M.; Ortiz, P.A.; Beierwaltes, W.H. Moderate (20%) fructose-enriched diet stimulates salt-sensitive hypertension with increased salt retention and decreased renal nitric oxide. *Physiol. Rep.* **2017**, *5*. [CrossRef]
7. Soncrant, T.; Komnenov, D.; Beierwaltes, W.H.; Chen, H.; Wu, M.; Rossi, N.F. Bilateral renal cryodenervation decreases arterial pressure and improves insulin sensitivity in fructose-fed Sprague-Dawley rats. *Am. J. Physiol. Regul. Integr. Comp. Physiol.* **2018**, *315*, R529–R538. [CrossRef]
8. Narain, A.; Kwok, C.S.; Mamas, M.A. Soft drinks and sweetened beverages and the risk of cardiovascular disease and mortality: A systematic review and meta-analysis. *Int J. Clin. Pract.* **2016**, *70*, 791–805. [CrossRef]

9. Lelis, D.F.; Andrade, J.M.O.; Almenara, C.C.P.; Broseguini-Filho, G.B.; Mill, J.G.; Baldo, M.P. High fructose intake and the route towards cardiometabolic diseases. *Life Sci.* **2020**, *259*, 118235. [CrossRef]
10. Eren, O.C.; Ortiz, A.; Afsar, B.; Covic, A.; Kuwabara, M.; Lanaspa, M.A.; Johnson, R.J.; Kanbay, M. Multilayered Interplay Between Fructose and Salt in Development of Hypertension. *Hypertension* **2019**, *73*, 265–272. [CrossRef] [PubMed]
11. Klein, A.V.; Kiat, H. The mechanisms underlying fructose-induced hypertension: A review. *J. Hypertens.* **2015**, *33*, 912–920. [CrossRef]
12. Perez-Pozo, S.E.; Schold, J.; Nakagawa, T.; Sanchez-Lozada, L.G.; Johnson, R.J.; Lillo, J.L. Excessive fructose intake induces the features of metabolic syndrome in healthy adult men: Role of uric acid in the hypertensive response. *Int. J. Obes. (Lond.)* **2010**, *34*, 454–461. [CrossRef]
13. Dhingra, R.; Sullivan, L.; Jacques, P.F.; Wang, T.J.; Fox, C.S.; Meigs, J.B.; D'Agostino, R.B.; Gaziano, J.M.; Vasan, R.S. Soft drink consumption and risk of developing cardiometabolic risk factors and the metabolic syndrome in middle-aged adults in the community. *Circulation* **2007**, *116*, 480–488. [CrossRef]
14. Fung, T.T.; Malik, V.; Rexrode, K.M.; Manson, J.E.; Willett, W.C.; Hu, F.B. Sweetened beverage consumption and risk of coronary heart disease in women. *Am. J. Clin. Nutr.* **2009**, *89*, 1037–1042. [CrossRef]
15. Aeberli, I.; Zimmermann, M.B.; Molinari, L.; Lehmann, R.; l'Allemand, D.; Spinas, G.A.; Berneis, K. Fructose intake is a predictor of LDL particle size in overweight schoolchildren. *Am. J. Clin. Nutr.* **2007**, *86*, 1174–1178. [CrossRef]
16. Park, Y.K.; Yetley, E.A. Intakes and food sources of fructose in the United States. *Am. J. Clin. Nutr.* **1993**, *58*, 737S–747S. [CrossRef]
17. Marriott, B.P.; Cole, N.; Lee, E. National estimates of dietary fructose intake increased from 1977 to 2004 in the United States. *J. Nutr.* **2009**, *139*, 1228S–1235S. [CrossRef]
18. Adriani, W.; Laviola, G. Windows of vulnerability to psychopathology and therapeutic strategy in the adolescent rodent model. *Behav. Pharmacol.* **2004**, *15*, 341–352. [CrossRef]
19. Sengupta, P. The Laboratory Rat: Relating Its Age With Human's. *Int. J. Prev. Med.* **2013**, *4*, 624–630. [PubMed]
20. Zicha, J.; Kunes, J. Ontogenetic aspects of hypertension development: Analysis in the rat. *Physiol. Rev.* **1999**, *79*, 1227–1282. [CrossRef] [PubMed]
21. Harrap, S.B.; Van der Merwe, W.M.; Griffin, S.A.; Macpherson, F.; Lever, A.F. Brief angiotensin converting enzyme inhibitor treatment in young spontaneously hypertensive rats reduces blood pressure long-term. *Hypertension* **1990**, *16*, 603–614. [CrossRef]
22. Rughani, A.; Friedman, J.E.; Tryggestad, J.B. Type 2 Diabetes in Youth: The Role of Early Life Exposures. *Curr. Diab. Rep.* **2020**, *20*, 45. [CrossRef]
23. Varlinskaya, E.I.; Spear, L.P. Social interactions in adolescent and adult Sprague-Dawley rats: Impact of social deprivation and test context familiarity. *Behav. Brain Res.* **2008**, *188*, 398–405. [CrossRef]
24. Coatney, R.W. Ultrasound imaging: Principles and applications in rodent research. *ILAR J.* **2001**, *42*, 233–247. [CrossRef]
25. Lindsey, M.L.; Kassiri, Z.; Virag, J.A.I.; de Castro Bras, L.E.; Scherrer-Crosbie, M. Guidelines for measuring cardiac physiology in mice. *Am. J. Physiol. Heart Circ. Physiol.* **2018**, *314*, H733–H752. [CrossRef]
26. O'Neill, W.C. Renal resistive index: A case of mistaken identity. *Hypertension* **2014**, *64*, 915–917. [CrossRef] [PubMed]
27. Komnenov, D.; Levanovich, P.E.; Perecki, N.; Chung, C.S.; Rossi, N.F. Aortic Stiffness and Diastolic Dysfunction in Sprague Dawley Rats Consuming Short-Term Fructose Plus High Salt Diet. *Integr. Blood Press Control* **2020**, *13*, 111–124. [CrossRef]
28. D'Angelo, G.; Elmarakby, A.A.; Pollock, D.M.; Stepp, D.W. Fructose feeding increases insulin resistance but not blood pressure in Sprague-Dawley rats. *Hypertension* **2005**, *46*, 806–811. [CrossRef]
29. Reaven, G.M.; Ho, H.; Hoffman, B.B. Attenuation of fructose-induced hypertension in rats by exercise training. *Hypertension* **1988**, *12*, 129–132. [CrossRef]
30. Johnson, M.D.; Zhang, H.Y.; Kotchen, T.A. Sucrose does not raise blood pressure in rats maintained on a low salt intake. *Hypertension* **1993**, *21*, 779–785. [CrossRef]
31. Paixao, A.D.; Alexander, B.T. How the kidney is impacted by the perinatal maternal environment to develop hypertension. *Biol. Reprod.* **2013**, *89*, 144. [CrossRef]
32. Gray, C.; Gardiner, S.M.; Elmes, M.; Gardner, D.S. Excess maternal salt or fructose intake programmes sex-specific, stress- and fructose-sensitive hypertension in the offspring. *Br. J. Nutr.* **2016**, *115*, 594–604. [CrossRef] [PubMed]
33. Ding, Y.; Lv, J.; Mao, C.; Zhang, H.; Wang, A.; Zhu, L.; Zhu, H.; Xu, Z. High-salt diet during pregnancy and angiotensin-related cardiac changes. *J. Hypertens.* **2010**, *28*, 1290–1297. [CrossRef]
34. Gray, C.; Al-Dujaili, E.A.; Sparrow, A.J.; Gardiner, S.M.; Craigon, J.; Welham, S.J.; Gardner, D.S. Excess maternal salt intake produces sex-specific hypertension in offspring: Putative roles for kidney and gastrointestinal sodium handling. *PLoS ONE* **2013**, *8*, e72682. [CrossRef]
35. Hocherl, K.; Endemann, D.; Kammerl, M.C.; Grobecker, H.F.; Kurtz, A. Cyclo-oxygenase-2 inhibition increases blood pressure in rats. *Br. J. Pharmacol.* **2002**, *136*, 1117–1126. [CrossRef]
36. Arashi, H.; Ogawa, H.; Yamaguchi, J.; Kawada-Watanabe, E.; Hagiwara, N. Impact of visit-to-visit variability and systolic blood pressure control on subsequent outcomes in hypertensive patients with coronary artery disease (from the HIJ-CREATE substudy). *Am. J. Cardiol.* **2015**, *116*, 236–242. [CrossRef]
37. Melgarejo, J.D.; Thijs, L.; Wei, D.M.; Bursztyn, M.; Yang, W.Y.; Li, Y.; Asayama, K.; Hansen, T.W.; Kikuya, M.; Ohkubo, T.; et al. Relative and Absolute Risk to Guide the Management of Pulse Pressure, an Age-Related Cardiovascular Risk Factor. *Am. J. Hypertens.* **2021**. [CrossRef]

38. Fyhrquist, F.; Metsarinne, K.; Tikkanen, I. Role of angiotensin II in blood pressure regulation and in the pathophysiology of cardiovascular disorders. *J. Hum. Hypertens.* **1995**, *9* (Suppl. 5), S19–S24.
39. Yang, N.; Hong, N.J.; Garvin, J.L. Dietary fructose enhances angiotensin II-stimulated Na(+) transport via activation of PKC-alpha in renal proximal tubules. *Am. J. Physiol. Ren. Physiol.* **2020**, *318*, F1513–F1519. [CrossRef]
40. Gonzalez-Vicente, A.; Cabral, P.D.; Hong, N.J.; Asirwatham, J.; Saez, F.; Garvin, J.L. Fructose reabsorption by rat proximal tubules: Role of Na(+)-linked cotransporters and the effect of dietary fructose. *Am. J. Physiol. Ren. Physiol.* **2019**, *316*, F473–F480. [CrossRef]
41. Gonzalez-Vicente, A.; Hong, N.J.; Yang, N.; Cabral, P.D.; Berthiaume, J.M.; Dominici, F.P.; Garvin, J.L. Dietary Fructose Increases the Sensitivity of Proximal Tubules to Angiotensin II in Rats Fed High-Salt Diets. *Nutrients* **2018**, *10*, 1244. [CrossRef]
42. Cabral, P.D.; Hong, N.J.; Hye Khan, M.A.; Ortiz, P.A.; Beierwaltes, W.H.; Imig, J.D.; Garvin, J.L. Fructose stimulates Na/H exchange activity and sensitizes the proximal tubule to angiotensin II. *Hypertension* **2014**, *63*, e68–e73. [CrossRef]
43. Ares, G.R.; Kassem, K.M.; Ortiz, P.A. Fructose acutely stimulates NKCC2 activity in rat thick ascending limbs by increasing surface NKCC2 expression. *Am. J. Physiol. Ren. Physiol.* **2019**, *316*, F550–F557. [CrossRef]
44. Katakam, P.V.; Ujhelyi, M.R.; Hoenig, M.E.; Miller, A.W. Endothelial dysfunction precedes hypertension in diet-induced insulin resistance. *Am. J. Physiol.* **1998**, *275*, R788–R792. [CrossRef]
45. Verma, S.; Bhanot, S.; McNeill, J.H. Effect of chronic endothelin blockade in hyperinsulinemic hypertensive rats. *Am. J. Physiol* **1995**, *269*, H2017–H2021. [CrossRef]
46. Nakagawa, T.; Hu, H.; Zharikov, S.; Tuttle, K.R.; Short, R.A.; Glushakova, O.; Ouyang, X.; Feig, D.I.; Block, E.R.; Herrera-Acosta, J.; et al. A causal role for uric acid in fructose-induced metabolic syndrome. *Am. J. Physiol. Ren. Physiol.* **2006**, *290*, F625–F631. [CrossRef]
47. Zenner, Z.P.; Gordish, K.L.; Beierwaltes, W.H. Free radical scavenging reverses fructose-induced salt-sensitive hypertension. *Integr. Blood Press Control* **2018**, *11*, 1–9. [CrossRef]
48. Humphrey, J.D.; Harrison, D.G.; Figueroa, C.A.; Lacolley, P.; Laurent, S. Central Artery Stiffness in Hypertension and Aging: A Problem With Cause and Consequence. *Circ. Res.* **2016**, *118*, 379–381. [CrossRef]
49. Gazhonova, V.E.; Zykova, A.S.; Chistyakov, A.A.; Roshchupkina, S.V.; Romanova, M.D.; Krasnova, T.N. Prognostic value of renal resistance index in estimating the progression of chronic kidney disease. *Ter. Arkh.* **2015**, *87*, 29–33. [CrossRef]
50. Radermacher, J.; Ellis, S.; Haller, H. Renal resistance index and progression of renal disease. *Hypertension* **2002**, *39*, 699–703. [CrossRef]
51. Parolini, C.; Noce, A.; Staffolani, E.; Giarrizzo, G.F.; Costanzi, S.; Splendiani, G. Renal resistive index and long-term outcome in chronic nephropathies. *Radiology* **2009**, *252*, 888–896. [CrossRef]
52. Mendonca, S.; Gupta, S. Resistive index predicts renal prognosis in chronic kidney disease. *Nephrol. Dial. Transplant.* **2010**, *25*, 644. [CrossRef] [PubMed]
53. Heine, G.H.; Rogacev, K.S.; Fliser, D.; Krumme, B. Renal resistive index and cardiovascular and renal outcomes in essential hypertension. *Hypertension* **2013**, *61*, e22. [CrossRef] [PubMed]
54. Doi, Y.; Iwashima, Y.; Yoshihara, F.; Kamide, K.; Hayashi, S.; Kubota, Y.; Nakamura, S.; Horio, T.; Kawano, Y. Renal resistive index and cardiovascular and renal outcomes in essential hypertension. *Hypertension* **2012**, *60*, 770–777. [CrossRef]
55. Tublin, M.E.; Bude, R.O.; Platt, J.F. Review. The resistive index in renal Doppler sonography: Where do we stand? *AJR Am. J. Roentgenol.* **2003**, *180*, 885–892. [CrossRef] [PubMed]
56. Ikee, R.; Kobayashi, S.; Hemmi, N.; Imakiire, T.; Kikuchi, Y.; Moriya, H.; Suzuki, S.; Miura, S. Correlation between the resistive index by Doppler ultrasound and kidney function and histology. *Am. J. Kidney Dis.* **2005**, *46*, 603–609. [CrossRef] [PubMed]
57. Boddi, M.; Cecioni, I.; Poggesi, L.; Fiorentino, F.; Olianti, K.; Berardino, S.; La Cava, G.; Gensini, G. Renal resistive index early detects chronic tubulointerstitial nephropathy in normo- and hypertensive patients. *Am. J. Nephrol.* **2006**, *26*, 16–21. [CrossRef]
58. Sugiura, T.; Nakamori, A.; Wada, A.; Fukuhara, Y. Evaluation of tubulointerstitial injury by Doppler ultrasonography in glomerular diseases. *Clin. Nephrol.* **2004**, *61*, 119–126. [CrossRef]
59. Riemer, K.; Rowland, E.M.; Leow, C.H.; Tang, M.X.; Weinberg, P.D. Determining Haemodynamic Wall Shear Stress in the Rabbit Aorta In Vivo Using Contrast-Enhanced Ultrasound Image Velocimetry. *Ann. Biomed. Eng.* **2020**, *48*, 1728–1739. [CrossRef]
60. Renna, N.F.; Lembo, C.; Diez, E.; Miatello, R.M. Role of Renin-Angiotensin system and oxidative stress on vascular inflammation in insulin resistence model. *Int. J. Hypertens.* **2013**, *2013*, 420979. [CrossRef]
61. Boron, W.F.; Boulpaep, E.L. *Medical Physiology*, 3rd ed.; Elsevier: Philadelphia, PA, USA, 2017; Chapter 23; pp. 533–555.
62. Tham, Y.K.; Bernardo, B.C.; Ooi, J.Y.; Weeks, K.L.; McMullen, J.R. Pathophysiology of cardiac hypertrophy and heart failure: Signaling pathways and novel therapeutic targets. *Arch. Toxicol.* **2015**, *89*, 1401–1438. [CrossRef]
63. Katz, D.H.; Beussink, L.; Sauer, A.J.; Freed, B.H.; Burke, M.A.; Shah, S.J. Prevalence, clinical characteristics, and outcomes associated with eccentric versus concentric left ventricular hypertrophy in heart failure with preserved ejection fraction. *Am. J. Cardiol.* **2013**, *112*, 1158–1164. [CrossRef] [PubMed]
64. Popovic, A.; Neskovic, N.; Marinkovic, J.; Lee, J.C.; Tan, M.; Thomas, J.D. Serial assessment of left ventricular chamber stiffness after acute myocardial infarction. *Am. J. Cardiol.* **1996**, *77*, 361–364. [CrossRef]
65. Satpathy, C.; Mishra, T.K.; Satpathy, R.; Satpathy, H.K.; Barone, E. Diagnosis and management of diastolic dysfunction and heart failure. *Am. Fam. Physician* **2006**, *73*, 841–846. [PubMed]
66. Huynh, K.; Bernardo, B.C.; McMullen, J.R.; Ritchie, R.H. Diabetic cardiomyopathy: Mechanisms and new treatment strategies targeting antioxidant signaling pathways. *Pharmacol. Ther.* **2014**, *142*, 375–415. [CrossRef] [PubMed]

67. Schannwell, C.M.; Schneppenheim, M.; Perings, S.; Plehn, G.; Strauer, B.E. Left ventricular diastolic dysfunction as an early manifestation of diabetic cardiomyopathy. *Cardiology* **2002**, *98*, 33–39. [CrossRef]
68. Zile, M.R.; Brutsaert, D.L. New concepts in diastolic dysfunction and diastolic heart failure: Part I: Diagnosis, prognosis, and measurements of diastolic function. *Circulation* **2002**, *105*, 1387–1393. [CrossRef]
69. Abdelhaffez, A.S.; Abd El-Aziz, E.A.; Tohamy, M.B.; Ahmed, A.M. N-acetyl cysteine can blunt metabolic and cardiovascular effects via down-regulation of cardiotrophin-1 in rat model of fructose-induced metabolic syndrome. *Arch. Physiol. Biochem.* **2021**, 1–16. [CrossRef]
70. Wang, S.; Wang, E.; Chen, Q.; Yang, Y.; Xu, L.; Zhang, X.; Wu, R.; Hu, X.; Wu, Z. Uncovering Potential lncRNAs and mRNAs in the Progression From Acute Myocardial Infarction to Myocardial Fibrosis to Heart Failure. *Front. Cardiovasc. Med.* **2021**, *8*, 664044. [CrossRef]
71. Galipeau, D.; Verma, S.; McNeill, J.H. Female rats are protected against fructose-induced changes in metabolism and blood pressure. *Am. J. Physiol. Heart Circ. Physiol.* **2002**, *283*, H2478–H2484. [CrossRef]
72. Verma, S.; Bhanot, S.; Yao, L.; McNeill, J.H. Vascular insulin resistance in fructose-hypertensive rats. *Eur. J. Pharmacol.* **1997**, *322*, R1–R2. [CrossRef]
73. Galipeau, D.M.; Yao, L.; McNeill, J.H. Relationship among hyperinsulinemia, insulin resistance, and hypertension is dependent on sex. *Am. J. Physiol. Heart Circ. Physiol.* **2002**, *283*, H562–H567. [CrossRef]
74. Song, D.; Arikawa, E.; Galipeau, D.M.; Yeh, J.N.; Battell, M.L.; Yuen, V.G.; McNeill, J.H. Chronic estrogen treatment modifies insulin-induced insulin resistance and hypertension in ovariectomized rats. *Am. J. Hypertens.* **2005**, *18*, 1189–1194. [CrossRef]
75. Vasudevan, H.; Xiang, H.; McNeill, J.H. Differential regulation of insulin resistance and hypertension by sex hormones in fructose-fed male rats. *Am. J. Physiol. Heart Circ. Physiol.* **2005**, *289*, H1335–H1342. [CrossRef]
76. Battiprolu, P.K.; Lopez-Crisosto, C.; Wang, Z.V.; Nemchenko, A.; Lavandero, S.; Hill, J.A. Diabetic cardiomyopathy and metabolic remodeling of the heart. *Life Sci.* **2013**, *92*, 609–615. [CrossRef]
77. Lamacchia, O.; Sorrentino, M.R. Diabetes Mellitus, Arterial Stiffness and Cardiovascular Disease: Clinical Implications and the Influence of SGLT2i. *Curr. Vasc. Pharmacol.* **2021**, *19*, 233–240. [CrossRef]
78. An, D.; Rodrigues, B. Role of changes in cardiac metabolism in development of diabetic cardiomyopathy. *Am. J. Physiol. Heart Circ. Physiol.* **2006**, *291*, H1489–H1506. [CrossRef] [PubMed]
79. Nikolajevic Starcevic, J.; Janic, M.; Sabovic, M. Molecular Mechanisms Responsible for Diastolic Dysfunction in Diabetes Mellitus Patients. *Int. J. Mol. Sci.* **2019**, *20*, 1197. [CrossRef] [PubMed]
80. Susic, D.; Varagic, J.; Ahn, J.; Frohlich, E.D. Crosslink breakers: A new approach to cardiovascular therapy. *Curr. Opin. Cardiol.* **2004**, *19*, 336–340. [CrossRef] [PubMed]
81. Nunes, S.; Soares, E.; Fernandes, J.; Viana, S.; Carvalho, E.; Pereira, F.C.; Reis, F. Early cardiac changes in a rat model of prediabetes: Brain natriuretic peptide overexpression seems to be the best marker. *Cardiovasc. Diabetol.* **2013**, *12*, 44. [CrossRef]
82. Drazner, M.H. The progression of hypertensive heart disease. *Circulation* **2011**, *123*, 327–334. [CrossRef]
83. Griffin, K.A. Hypertensive Kidney Injury and the Progression of Chronic Kidney Disease. *Hypertension* **2017**, *70*, 687–694. [CrossRef] [PubMed]

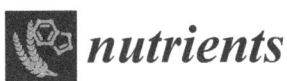

Article

Effects of Elaidic Acid on HDL Cholesterol Uptake Capacity

Takuya Iino [1,2], Ryuji Toh [3,*], Manabu Nagao [3], Masakazu Shinohara [4,5], Amane Harada [2], Katsuhiro Murakami [2], Yasuhiro Irino [2], Makoto Nishimori [1], Sachiko Yoshikawa [1], Yutaro Seto [1], Tatsuro Ishida [1] and Ken-ichi Hirata [1,3]

[1] Division of Cardiovascular Medicine, Graduate School of Medicine, Kobe University, Kobe 650-0017, Japan; iino@med.kobe-u.ac.jp (T.I.); mnishi.mail@gmail.com (M.N.); sachi.ys1228@gmail.com (S.Y.); y.seto0318@gmail.com (Y.S.); ishida@med.kobe-u.ac.jp (T.I.); hiratak@med.kobe-u.ac.jp (K.-i.H.)

[2] Central Research Laboratories, Sysmex Corporation, 4-4-4 Takatsukadai, Nishi-ku, Kobe 651-2271, Japan; Harada.Amane@sysmex.co.jp (A.H.); Murakami.Katsuhiro@sysmex.co.jp (K.M.); Irino.Yasuhiro@sysmex.co.jp (Y.I.)

[3] Division of Evidence-Based Laboratory Medicine, Graduate School of Medicine, Kobe University, Kobe 650-0017, Japan; mnagao@med.kobe-u.ac.jp

[4] Division of Epidemiology, Graduate School of Medicine, Kobe University, Kobe 650-0017, Japan; mashino@med.kobe-u.ac.jp

[5] The Integrated Center for Mass Spectrometry, Graduate School of Medicine, Kobe University, Kobe 650-0017, Japan

* Correspondence: rtoh@med.kobe-u.ac.jp

Abstract: Recently we established a cell-free assay to evaluate "cholesterol uptake capacity (CUC)" as a novel concept for high-density lipoprotein (HDL) functionality and demonstrated the feasibility of CUC for coronary risk stratification, although its regulatory mechanism remains unclear. HDL fluidity affects cholesterol efflux, and trans fatty acids (TFA) reduce lipid membrane fluidity when incorporated into phospholipids (PL). This study aimed to clarify the effect of TFA in HDL-PL on CUC. Serum was collected from 264 patients after coronary angiography or percutaneous coronary intervention to measure CUC and elaidic acid levels in HDL-PL, and in vitro analysis using reconstituted HDL (rHDL) was used to determine the HDL-PL mechanism affecting CUC. CUC was positively associated with HDL-PL levels but negatively associated with the proportion of elaidic acid in HDL-PL (elaidic acid in HDL-PL/HDL-PL ratio). Increased elaidic acid-phosphatidylcholine (PC) content in rHDL exhibited no change in particle size or CUC compared to rHDL containing oleic acid in PC. Recombinant human lecithin-cholesterol acyltransferase (LCAT) enhanced CUC, and LCAT-dependent enhancement of CUC and LCAT-dependent cholesterol esterification were suppressed in rHDL containing elaidic acid in PC. Therefore, CUC is affected by HDL-PL concentration, HDL-PL acyl group composition, and LCAT-dependent cholesterol esterification. Elaidic acid precipitated an inhibition of cholesterol uptake and maturation of HDL; therefore, modulation of HDL-PL acyl groups could improve CUC.

Keywords: high-density lipoprotein (HDL); cholesterol uptake capacity (CUC); phospholipids (PL); trans-fatty acids (TFA); elaidic acid; lecithin-cholesterol acyltransferase (LCAT)

1. Introduction

High-density lipoprotein (HDL) is a multifunctional lipoprotein that protects against atherosclerosis. Although the detailed mechanisms are yet to be elucidated, a key function of HDL to protect cardiovascular events is suggested to be the efflux of cholesterol from macrophages in the arterial wall, which could be measured as cholesterol efflux capacity (CEC).

Previous studies have demonstrated a negative correlation between CEC and the probability of coronary artery disease (CAD) independent of HDL cholesterol (HDL-C) concentration [1–3]. However, since CEC assays require radiolabeled cholesterol and cultured cells and time consuming procedures [4,5], application of CEC in clinical settings is challenging. To overcome the technical limitations related to CEC, we recently established a simple, high-throughput, cell-free assay system to evaluate cholesterol uptake capacity (CUC) as a novel concept for HDL functionality. We have reported an inverse association between CUC and the recurrence rate of coronary lesions after revascularization in patients with optimal control of low-density lipoprotein cholesterol (LDL-C) concentrations [6,7]. However, the regulatory mechanism of CUC remains unclear.

Several studies have shown that the ability of HDL to accept cellular free cholesterol is related to the amount of phospholipids (PL) present in the particle [8,9], and that PL containing unsaturated fatty acids in their acyl groups increase the fluidity of the HDL surface and improve cholesterol efflux when incorporated into HDL [10]. In addition, we recently reported that oral administration of purified eicosapentaenoic acid (EPA) generates EPA-rich HDL particles, which exhibit cardioprotective properties via the production of anti-inflammatory lipid metabolites and an increase in cholesterol efflux [11,12]. These results indicate the importance of acyl groups of PL in HDL functionality.

Trans-fatty acids (TFA) are unsaturated fatty acids with at least one unsaturated double bond in the trans structure, whose excess intake is considered to be associated with an increased risk of cardiovascular disease (CVD) [13–17]. Previous studies have shown that TFA taken orally are incorporated into PL in plasma [18], where they reduce the fluidity of lipid membranes [19]. Considering that PL are the major lipid component of HDL [20], these results indicate the possibility that TFA are incorporated into the PL of HDL and affect its functionality. However, the relationship between CUC and TFA incorporated into HDL phospholipids (HDL-PL) has not yet been investigated. Therefore, the present study aimed to clarify the effect of TFA in HDL-PL on CUC.

2. Materials and Methods

2.1. Subjects

The Kobe Cardiovascular Marker Investigation (CMI) registry is a single-center registry of patients referred to Kobe University Hospital with cardiovascular disease, which is used to identify blood-based biomarkers that are useful in predicting cardiovascular disease. The study protocol was in accordance with the ethical guidelines of the 1975 Declaration of Helsinki. The study was approved by the Ethics Review Committee at Kobe University (Japan) and was registered in the UMIN Clinical Trials Registry (identification number 000030297). Written informed consent was obtained from all patients prior to enrollment in the study.

Serum samples were collected from patients who underwent coronary angiography (CAG) or percutaneous coronary intervention (PCI) and stored at 80 °C until measurement. The inclusion criteria for this study were patients with a history of PCI and follow-up CAG with or without revascularization between July 2015 and February 2019. Exclusion criteria were patients who did not have frozen serum samples for any reason.

2.2. Preparation of the apoB-Depleted Serum

Serum samples were thawed on ice and incubated with the same volume of 22% polyethylene glycol (PEG) 4000 to remove apolipoprotein B (apoB)-containing lipoproteins. Briefly, each serum sample was mixed with a PEG solution and kept at room temperature for 20 min. The samples were then centrifuged at $860\times g$ for 15 min to precipitate all apoB-containing lipoproteins, and the supernatant was collected as apoB-depleted serum. A previous study that used gel filtration chromatography showed that cholesterol and PL colocalized in the same fraction as HDL in apoB-depleted serum [21]. Therefore, we used apoB-depleted serum for the HDL-PL analysis.

2.3. Clinical Variables

Serum levels of hemoglobin A1c (HbA1c), triglyceride (TG), total cholesterol (TC), LDL-C, HDL-C, and high-density lipoprotein triglyceride (HDL-TG) were measured using a standard assay at the Clinical Laboratory of Kobe University Hospital. HDL-PL levels were assessed by measuring apoB-depleted serum diluted eight times in phosphate-buffered saline (PBS) at SRL, Inc. (Hachioji, Tokyo, Japan) and calibrated using three-fold serially diluted pooled serum.

2.4. CUC Assay

The development of the CUC assay has been described previously [6,7]. In this study, the assay principle was applied to the HI-1000™ system (Sysmex, Kobe, Japan), which is a fully automated immunoassay system for research applications. In brief, 5 µL of apoB-depleted serum was diluted in a buffer containing PBS and 0.2% R1 reagent of the HDL-C Reagent KL "kokusai" (Sysmex, Kobe, Japan) 200 times, and 10 µL of the diluted apoB-depleted serum was incubated with 90 µL of 1 µM biotin-PEG-labeled cholesterol (the preparation method is described in Appendix A) in reaction buffer (PBS containing 11% glycerol, 1.1% Pluronic F-68 (Thermo Fisher Scientific, Inc., Waltham, MA, USA), 0.11 mM methyl-β-cyclodextrin (Merck KGaA, Darmstadt, Germany), 0.055% liposome (Nippon fine chemical, Tokyo, Japan), 0.0047% nonion-K230 (NOF, Tokyo, Japan), 0.37% SF08 (NOF, Tokyo, Japan), and 0.009% oleamide (Kao, Tokyo, Japan)) at 37 °C for 1 min. Serum HDL was captured by an anti-apolipoprotein A1 (apoA1) mouse monoclonal antibody clone 8E10 (the preparation method is described in Appendix A) coated on magnetic particles at 37 °C for 6 min. After washing the particles with wash buffer (HISCL™ line washing solution containing 0.1% Pluronic F-68 and 138 mM sodium chloride), 100 µL of alkaline phosphatase-conjugated streptavidin (Vector Laboratories, Burlingame, CA, USA) in dilution buffer (0.1 M TEA (pH 7.5) containing 10 mg/mL BSA, 5 mg/mL Casein Na, 1 mM $MgCl_2$, and 0.1 mM $ZnCl_2$) was added and incubated at 37 °C for 10 min. After washing the particles with wash buffer, the chemiluminescent substrate was added and incubated at 42 °C for 5 min, and chemiluminescence was measured as a count. The CUC assay was standardized using the pooled serum.

2.5. Measurement of Elaidic Acid Incorporated into HDL Phospholipids

One hundred microliters of 50 µM 1,2-dinonadecanoyl-sn-glycero-3-phosphocholine (19:0 PC; Merck KGaA, Darmstadt, Germany) were added to 200 µL of apoB-depleted serum as an internal standard, and total lipids were extracted using the Bligh and Dyer method as described previously [22] and applied to InertSep SI columns (GL Sciences Inc., Tokyo, Japan). The columns were then washed with 3 mL of chloroform and 3 mL of acetone. PL were eluted from the columns using 6 mL of methanol, dried under N_2, and methylated with a commercially available kit (Nacalai Tesque, Kyoto, Japan) according to the manufacturer's protocol. The concentrations of methylated elaidic acid were measured using gas chromatography-mass spectrometry (GC-MS). The GC-MS conditions used for the measurements in this study were described in a previous study [13], except that the split-less injection mode was adopted to increase the sensitivity, and each value was standardized using pooled serum.

2.6. Preparation of rHDL

The rHDL particles were prepared using a previously described sodium cholate dialysis method [12,23]. In brief, the required amounts of 1-palmitoyl-2-oleoyl-sn-glycero-3-phosphocholine (POPC) (Merck KGaA, Darmstadt, Germany), 1,2-dioleoyl-sn-glycero-3-phosphocholine (DOPC) (Merck KGaA, Darmstadt, Germany), or 1,2-dielaidoyl-sn-glycero-3-phosphocholine (elaidic acid PC) (Merck KGaA, Darmstadt, Germany), and cholesterol (FUJIFILM Wako Pure Chemical Corporation, Osaka, Japan) were mixed and dried under an N_2 gas stream. The dried mixture was dissolved in tris(hydroxymethyl)aminomethane (Tris)-buffered saline (TBS; 8.2 mmol/L Tris-HCl, 150 mmol/L NaCl, pH 8.0) and supplemented with 19 mmol/L sodium deoxycholate until the solution was clear. ApoA1 from human plasma (Merck KGaA, Darmstadt, Germany) was added to the solution to make a final phosphatidylcholine (PC)–cholesterol–apoA1 molar ratio of 30:2:1. The mixture was incubated at 37 °C for 1 h and dialyzed against TBS for three days to remove sodium deoxycholate. The protein concentration was measured using the Bradford protein assay. The samples were subjected to non-denaturing 4–20% gradient polyacrylamide gel (Bio-Rad, Hercules, CA, USA) electrophoresis and stained with Coomassie Brilliant Blue to visualize the rHDL particles. Particle size was assigned by comparison with protein standards using a high molecular weight calibration kit (GE Healthcare, Madison, WI, USA).

2.7. CUC Assay for rHDL

rHDL was diluted in buffer to obtain a final apoA1 concentration of 1 µg/mL, and the CUC assay was performed with the HI-1000^{TM} system as described above. To evaluate the effects of lecithin-cholesterol acyltransferase (LCAT) on the CUC assay, recombinant human LCAT (rhLCAT) (Sino Biological Inc., Beijing, China) or rhLCAT preincubated with 2 mM N-ethylmaleimide (NEM) (FUJIFILM Wako Pure Chemical Corporation, Osaka, Japan) at 30 °C for 30 min were mixed with rHDL to make a final rhLCAT–apoA1 molar ratio of 1.5:1 or 4.2:1, respectively, and incubated at 37 °C for 5 min. The samples were then diluted in buffer to obtain a final apoA1 concentration of 1 µg/mL, and the CUC assay was performed. The quantification of apoA1 was conducted using the HI-1000^{TM} system and standardized using pooled serum. Briefly, an alkaline phosphatase-conjugated anti-apoA1 mouse monoclonal antibody clone P1A5 (the preparation method is described in Appendix A) was added to rHDL captured by an anti-apoA1 mouse monoclonal antibody (8E10)-coated on magnetic particles and incubated at 37 °C for 10 min. After washing the particles with wash buffer, the chemiluminescent substrate was added and incubated at 42 °C for 5 min, and chemiluminescence was measured as a count. To improve inter- and intra-assay precision, the CUC per apoA1 value was used for CUC analysis of rHDL.

2.8. Fluorescence-Based Assay for LCAT Activity

A fluorescence-based assay for LCAT activity was developed according to a previous study [24]. The rHDL particles containing POPC or elaidic acid-PC, BODIPY-cholesterol (Avanti Polar Lipids, Alabaster, AL, USA), and apoA1 in a ratio of 30:2:1 were prepared and used as proteoliposome substrates. The samples were subjected to non-denaturing 4–20% gradient polyacrylamide gel (Bio-Rad, Hercules, CA, USA) electrophoresis and analyzed with a ChemiDoc Touch MP (Bio-Rad, Hercules, CA, USA) set at 488 nm for excitation and 520 nm for emission to detect BODIPY-cholesterol. The same gel was stained with Coomassie Brilliant Blue to visualize the rHDL particles.

The rhLCAT or rhLCAT preincubated with 2 mM NEM at 30 °C for 30 min was mixed with the proteoliposome substrates to make a final rhLCAT:apoA1 molar ratio of 0.5:1, and incubated at 37 °C for 10–90 min. The lipids were extracted from the samples, dissolved in 30 µL of chloroform, and applied to a thin-layer chromatography (TLC) silica gel 60 plate (Merck KGaA, Darmstadt, Germany), which was then placed into a closed glass tank and saturated with a developing solvent (petroleum ether, diethyl ether, and acetic acid in mole portions of 230:60:3). After 25 min, the TLC plate was removed from the tank and cholesterol spots and esterified cholesterol spots were detected using a ChemiDoc Touch MP set at 488 nm for excitation and 520 nm for emission. For quantitative analysis of cholesterol esterification rate, the TLC plate was exposed for 0.2 s and the fluorescence intensities of both cholesterol spots and esterified cholesterol spots were quantified by densitometry analysis using ImageJ® software (NIH, Bethesda, MD, USA). The cholesterol esterification rate was calculated using the following formula:

% Cholesterol esterification rate = (Fluorescence intensities of esterified BODIPY-cholesterol spots derived from each rHDL/Fluorescence intensities of BODIPY-cholesterol spots derived from rHDL without addition of rhLCAT) × 100.

For visual inspection, exposure time for detecting BODIPY-cholesterol and esterified BODIPY-cholesterol spots were set to 0.2 and 3.0 s, respectively.

2.9. Statistics

Statistical analyses of clinical subjects were performed using Stata 16.1 (StataCorp LLC, College Station, TX, USA), and for rHDL, the GraphPad Prism software version 8.4.3 (GraphPad Software, Inc., San Diego, CA, USA). Categorical variables were expressed as numbers and percentages, and the p value for differences between two groups was determined using the Chi-square test. Continuous variables were expressed as mean ± standard deviation (SD), unless otherwise specified. The p value for differences between two groups was determined by an unpaired Student's t-test or the Mann–Whitney test according to the data distribution and normality. Differences between multiple groups were determined by one-way ANOVA with Tukey's or Dunnett's multiple comparisons test, as applicable. The relationships between the two numerical variables were investigated using a simple linear regression analysis. We report Spearman's rho with corresponding p values. Statistical significance was set at $p < 0.05$.

3. Results

3.1. Baseline Patient Characteristics

From the Kobe CMI registry between July 2015 and February 2019, we enrolled 264 patients based on the inclusion and exclusion criteria. The baseline patient characteristics and laboratory data are shown in Table 1.

Table 1. Baseline patient characteristics and laboratory data.

Variables	n = 264
Age	70.8 ± 9.3
Male, n (%)	210 (79.5)
Hypertension, n (%)	204 (77.3)
Dyslipidemia, n (%)	221 (83.7)
Diabetes, n (%)	119 (45.1)
Smoking history, n (%)	180 (68.4)
Statin, n (%)	233 (88.2)
Laboratory data	
HbA1c (%)	6.4 ± 1.0
TG (mg/dL)	128.8 ± 71.2
TC (mg/dL)	146.8 ± 31.2
LDL-C (mg/dL)	82.1 ± 26.3
HDL-C (mg/dL)	46.1 ± 12.6
CUC (A.U.)	94.8 ± 20.5
ApoA1 (mg/dL)	118.0 ± 19.3
HDL-PL (mg/dL)	78.0 ± 26.6
HDL-TG (mg/dL)	13.6 ± 6.6
Elaidic acid in HDL-PL (μM)	1.1 ± 0.50

Values are presented as mean ± SD. HbA1c, hemoglobin A1c; TG, triglyceride; TC, total cholesterol; LDL-C, low-density lipoprotein cholesterol; HDL-C, high-density lipoprotein cholesterol; CUC, cholesterol uptake capacity; ApoA1, apolipoprotein A1; HDL-PL, high-density lipoprotein phospholipid; HDL-TG, high-density lipoprotein triglyceride; A.U., arbitrary units.

More than 80% of the patients were receiving statin therapy, and achieved a mean LDL-C level of less than 100 mg/dL, which is the goal for secondary prevention of coronary artery disease (CAD) in Japan [25]. The patients in the revascularization (Rev.(+) group had a significantly higher incidence of diabetes than patients without revascularization (Rev.(−)). Conversely, CUC and HDL-PL levels were significantly higher in the Rev.(−) patients than those in the Rev.(+) group. Elaidic acid levels in HDL-PL also tended to be higher in the Rev.(−) group than in the Rev.(+) group, although this trend was not statistically significant (Supplemental Tables S1 and S2).

3.2. The Proportion of Elaidic Acid in HDL-PL Inversely Correlates with CUC

As a first step towards understanding the effect of TFA in HDL-PL on CUC, we assessed the relationship between CUC and HDL-PL and confirmed that CUC was positively associated with HDL-PL levels (rS = 0.906, $p < 0.001$) (Figure 1A). Though CUC was also positively associated with apoA1 levels (rS = 0.683, $p < 0.001$) (Figure S1A), the value of correlation coefficient was smaller than that of HDL-PL levels, suggesting that the HDL-PL level is an important factor in determining CUC.

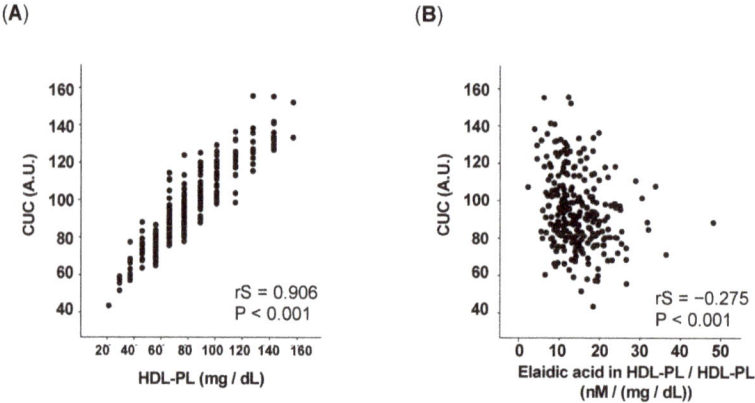

Figure 1. Correlations between CUC and the following: (**A**) HDL-PL levels (rS = 0.906, $p < 0.001$), (**B**) elaidic acid in HDL PL/HDL-PL ratio (rS = −0.275, $p < 0.001$). CUC, cholesterol uptake capacity; A.U., arbitrary units; HDL-PL, high-density lipoprotein phospholipid.

To analyze the effect of TFA incorporated into HDL-PL on CUC, we evaluated the relationship between CUC and elaidic acid in HDL-PL and found that although there was a positive correlation (Figure S1B); CUC was negatively associated with the proportion of elaidic acid in the HDL-PL/HDL-PL ratio (rS = −0.275, $p < 0.001$) (Figure 1B). By contrast, though oleic acid, a cis analogue of elaidic acid, in HDL-PL also correlated positively with CUC (Figure S1C), no significant relationship was noted between CUC and the proportion of oleic acid in HDL-PL (Figure S1D). These results indicate the possibility that elaidic acid has a negative effect on CUC when incorporated into HDL-PL.

3.3. LCAT-Dependent Enhancement of CUC Is Suppressed in rHDL Containing Elaidic Acid-PC

To investigate the effects of elaidic acid in HDL-PL on HDL size and functionality, discoidal rHDL containing various molar percentages of POPC and elaidic acid-PC (0–100% of total PC) were prepared and particle size and CUC were assessed. Native PAGE analysis showed that particle sizes did not differ significantly between rHDLs (Figure 2A).

Similarly, contrary to our expectation, the elaidic acid-PC content in rHDL did not affect CUC (Figure 2B), although these results might have been due to the limitations of CUC analysis using only rHDL.

Under physiological conditions, LCAT is known to bind discoidal small HDLs (pre-β-HDL) [26,27] and is important for HDL maturation [28]. In peripheral tissues, free cholesterol effluxes from cells by the ATP-binding cassette transporter A1 (ABCA1) to pre-β-HDL and is esterified by LCAT. Due to their hydrophobic chemical properties, cholesterol esters (CE) move to the core of the HDL [29], making it larger and more spherical mature. Recently, it has been reported that rhLCAT increased CE and enhanced cholesterol efflux and the maturation of HDL in vivo [30]. Therefore, we hypothesized that the addition of rhLCAT to rHDL would enable CUC analysis under near-physiological conditions.

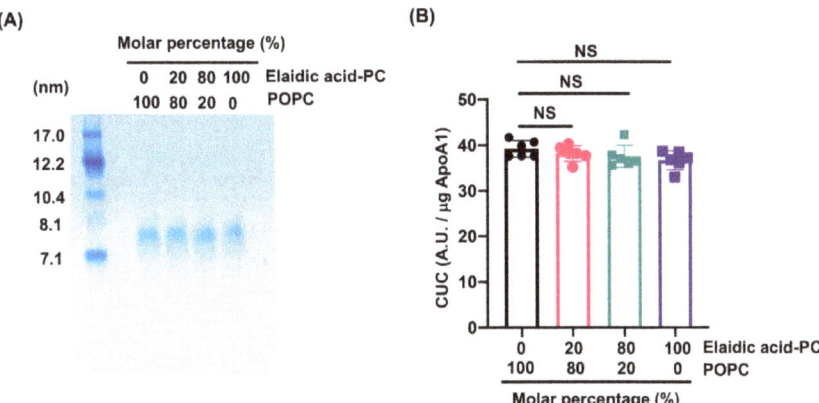

Figure 2. Elaidic acid-PC contents in rHDL do not affect particle size and CUC. (**A**) rHDL containing different POPC and elaidic acid-PC molar percentages was prepared and native polyacrylamide gel electrophoresis (PAGE) analysis was performed in a 4–20% polyacrylamide gel to assess the particle size. Standard proteins of known hydrodynamic diameters were used for this analysis. Samples (1.0 μg proteins) were separated by non-denaturing gel electrophoresis and stained with Coomassie Brilliant Blue. (**B**) rHDL containing different POPC and elaidic acid-PC molar percentages was prepared and CUC assay was performed. Values are expressed as the mean ± SD (n = 6). CUC, cholesterol uptake capacity; A.U., arbitrary units; NS, not significant. Data analyzed by one-way ANOVA with Dunnett's multiple comparisons test.

To investigate the effects of LCAT on CUC, rHDL containing POPC was prepared and the CUC assay was performed in the presence of rhLCAT or rhLCAT pre-incubated with NEM, which inhibits LCAT activity [31–34]. The addition of rhLCAT to rHDL significantly enhanced CUC, and LCAT-dependent enhancement of CUC was suppressed by NEM (Figure 3A).

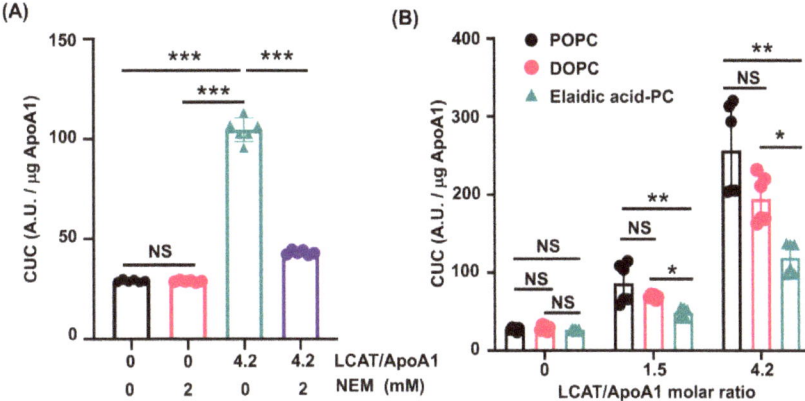

Figure 3. LCAT-dependent enhancement of CUC is suppressed in rHDL containing elaidic acid-PC. (**A**) rHDL containing POPC was prepared and a CUC assay was performed in the presence of rhLCAT or rhLCAT pre-incubated with NEM. Values are expressed as the mean ± SD (n = 6). LCAT, lecithin cholesterol acyltransferase; apoA1, apolipoprotein A1; NEM, N-ethylmaleimide; CUC, cholesterol uptake capacity; A.U., arbitrary units. *** $p < 0.001$. NS, not significant. Data analyzed by one-way ANOVA with Tukey's multiple comparisons test. (**B**) rHDL containing POPC, DOPC, and elaidic acid-PC was prepared and a CUC assay was performed in the presence of rhLCAT. Values are expressed as the mean ± SD (n = 6). * $p < 0.05$, ** $p < 0.01$. NS, not significant. Data analyzed by one-way ANOVA with Dunnett's multiple comparisons test.

Next, to investigate the effects of elaidic acid in HDL-PL on CUC in the presence of LCAT, rHDL containing POPC, DOPC, and elaidic acid-PC were prepared and the CUC assay was performed in the presence of rhLCAT. Although PL contain saturated fatty acids mainly in the sn1 position [35–37], we used a PC containing elaidic acid in both the sn1 and sn2 positions as elaidic acid-PC. To confirm the effect of sn1 substitution by monounsaturated fatty acids, DOPC, which contains oleic acid in both the sn1 and sn2 positions, and POPC, which contains palmitic acid in the sn1 position and oleic acid in the sn2 position, were used as controls. Although rhLCAT-dependent enhancement of CUC was observed in all rHDLs, the CUC of rHDL containing elaidic acid-PC was significantly lower than that of rHDL containing POPC or DOPC (Figure 3B). These findings indicate that LCAT plays a crucial role in the enhancement of CUC, and elaidic acid has a negative effect on CUC in the presence of LCAT.

3.4. LCAT-Dependent Cholesterol Esterification Is Suppressed in rHDL Containing Elaidic Acid-PC

Previous studies have shown that conversion of free cholesterol on HDL to CE by LCAT increases the capacity of HDL to remove additional cholesterol and maintains the gradient for cholesterol efflux from cells [29,30]. Therefore, we speculated that elaidic acid in HDL-PL inhibited LCAT-dependent cholesterol esterification on HDL and affected CUC. To evaluate LCAT-dependent cholesterol esterification, a fluorescence-based assay for LCAT activity was developed according to a previous study [24]. First, we prepared rHDL containing both BODIPY-cholesterol and POPC as a proteoliposome substrate and confirmed that the fluorescent signal was detected in the same size as rHDL by native PAGE analysis (Figure 4A).

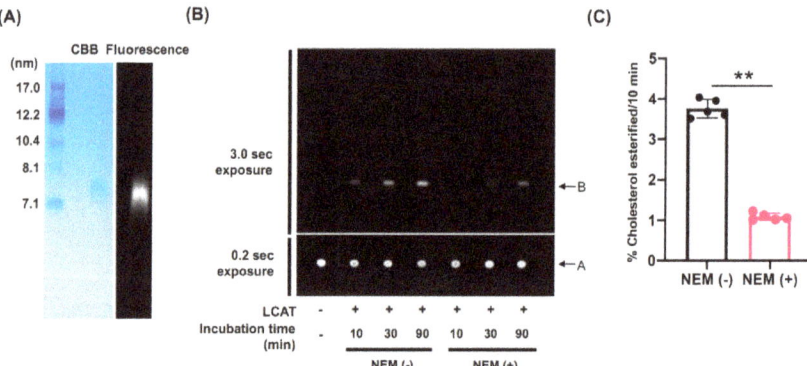

Figure 4. Development of a fluorescence-based assay for LCAT activity. (**A**) rHDL containing both BODIPY-cholesterol and POPC was prepared and native PAGE analysis was performed in a 4–20% polyacrylamide gel. Standard proteins of known hydrodynamic diameters were used for the analysis. Samples (1.0 µg proteins) were separated by non-denaturing gel electrophoresis and stained with Coomassie Brilliant Blue (left). The same Native PAGE gel was analyzed with a ChemiDoc Touch MP (Bio-Rad) set at 488 nm for excitation and 520 nm for emission (right). (**B**) rhLCAT or rhLCAT pre-incubated with NEM was incubated with rHDL containing BODIPY-cholesterol and POPC for 10–90 min at 37 °C. The extracted lipids were dissolved in 30 µL of chloroform and applied to the TLC plate. The TLC plate was placed into a closed glass tank, saturated by a developing solvent (petroleum ether, diethyl ether, and acetic acid in mole portions of 230:60:3). After 25 min, the plate was removed and the cholesterol spots (Position A) and esterified cholesterol spots (Position B) were detected using a ChemiDoc Touch MP set at 488 nm for excitation and 520 nm for emission. In order to visualize spots clearly, cholesterol spots were exposed for 0.2 s and esterified cholesterol spots were exposed for 3.0 s. (**C**) The TLC plate was exposed for 0.2 s and cholesterol spots and esterified cholesterol spots were quantified by densitometry analysis using ImageJ® software. Cholesterol esterification rate was calculated as the percentage of cholesterol esterified during HDL incubation at 37 °C in 10 min. Values are expressed as the mean ± SD ($n = 5$). ** $p < 0.01$. Data analyzed by unpaired Mann–Whitney test.

Second, rhLCAT or rhLCAT pre-incubated with NEM was incubated with rHDL for 10–90 min, both BODIPY-cholesterol and esterified BODIPY-cholesterol were separated by TLC, and fluorescent signals were detected. Fluorescent intensities of esterified BODIPY-cholesterol increased depending on the incubation time in the presence of rhLCAT, and this trend was suppressed by pre-incubation of rhLCAT with NEM (Figure 4B). Quantitative analysis also showed that the LCAT-dependent cholesterol esterification rate was suppressed by NEM (Figure 4C). We concluded from these results that the fluorescence activity assay for LCAT developed properly.

Finally, to evaluate the effect of elaidic acid in HDL-PL on LCAT-dependent cholesterol esterification, rHDL containing both BODIPY-cholesterol and POPC or elaidic acid-PC were prepared as proteoliposome substrates and a fluorescence activity assay for LCAT was performed. Although the fluorescent intensities of esterified BODIPY-cholesterol increased depending on the incubation time in the presence of LCAT in both rHDLs (Figure 5A), the cholesterol esterification rate of rHDL containing elaidic acid-PC was significantly lower than that of rHDL containing POPC (Figure 5B), demonstrating that elaidic acid suppresses esterification of cholesterol on HDL when incorporated into HDL-PL.

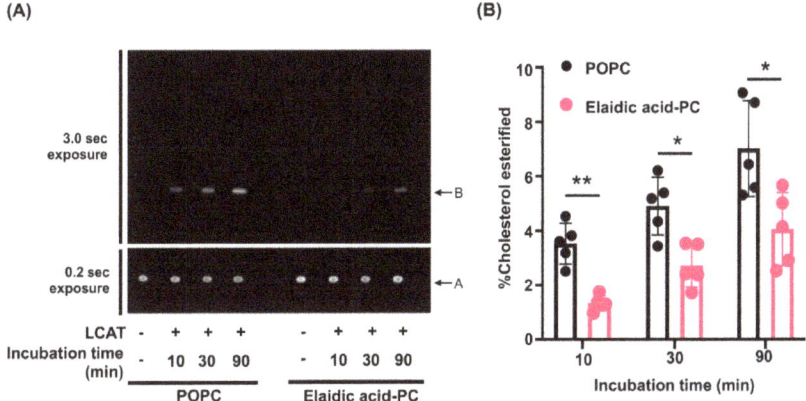

Figure 5. LCAT-dependent cholesterol esterification is suppressed in rHDL containing elaidic acid-PC. (**A**) rHDL containing both BODIPY-cholesterol and POPC or elaidic acid-PC were prepared and incubated with rhLCAT for 10–90 min at 37 °C. The extracted lipids were dissolved in 30 µL of chloroform and applied to the TLC plate. The TLC plate was placed into a closed glass tank, saturated by a developing solvent (petroleum ether, diethyl ether, and acetic acid in mole portions of 230:60:3). After 25 min, the plate was removed and the cholesterol spots (Position A) and esterified cholesterol spots (Position B) were detected using a ChemiDoc Touch MP. In order to visualize the spots clearly, cholesterol spots were exposed for 0.2 sec and esterified cholesterol spots were exposed for 3.0 sec. (**B**) The TLC plate was exposed for 0.2 sec and cholesterol spots and esterified cholesterol spots were quantified by densitometry analysis using ImageJ® software. Cholesterol esterification rate was calculated as the percentage of cholesterol esterified during HDL incubation at 37 °C for, 10–90 min. Values are expressed as the mean ± SD (n = 5). * $p < 0.05$ ** $p < 0.01$. Data analyzed by unpaired Mann–Whitney test.

4. Discussion

In this study, we demonstrated that CUC, a novel indicator of HDL functionality, was inversely associated with the proportion of elaidic acid in HDL-PL. In vitro analysis using rHDL showed that rhLCAT enhanced CUC, and LCAT-dependent enhancement of CUC was suppressed in rHDL containing elaidic acid in PC compared to rHDL containing oleic acid, a cis analogue of elaidic acid. Moreover, we found that LCAT-dependent cholesterol esterification was also suppressed by elaidic acid.

PL are major components of the HDL lipidome, accounting for 40–60% of total HDL lipids, followed by cholesteryl esters (30–40%), triglycerides (5–12%), and free cholesterol (5–10%) [20]. In the present study, we found that HDL-PL levels were strongly significantly correlated with CUC, which agrees with previous studies that showed a significantly positive correlation between CEC and HDL-PL levels [38]. In vitro analysis using rHDL also showed that CEC at a fixed rHDL protein concentration increased in parallel with increasingly enriched PL [39]. Since cholesterol interacts with PL [40], the latter are indispensable components for maintaining cholesterol in lipid membranes. We believe that our results reflect the intrinsic mechanism of the affinity between PL and cholesterol.

Previously, we showed that serum elaidic acid levels were elevated in middle-aged patients with CAD and/or metabolic syndrome in Japan [13]. We also showed that elevated serum elaidic acid levels were associated with the incidence of target vessel revascularization (TLR) in the same-age Japanese generation with CAD [14]. Dietary TFA are reported to be associated with increased LDL-C and TG, as well as reduced HDL-C [41], suggesting that the adverse effects of TFA on lipoprotein quantity and function may contribute to the increase in CVD events. Nevertheless, the effects of TFA on HDL functionality have not been completely elucidated.

In this study, both CUC and HDL-PL levels were significantly higher in the Rev.(−) group than in the Rev.(+) group. Accompanied by the increase in HDL-PL levels, the elaidic acid levels in HDL-PL also tended to be higher in the Rev.(−) group than in the Rev.(+) group. However, this trend was not statistically significant. To investigate the effect of the elaidic acid composition of HDL-PL on CUC, we examined the relationship between the proportion of elaidic acid in HDL-PL (elaidic acid in HDL-PL/HDL-PL ratio) and CUC, and found a negative correlation. By contrast, oleic acid, a cis analogue of elaidic acid, showed no such relationship. These results suggest that not only the amount of PL but also the composition of PL is a factor in determining CUC, and that the increased proportion of elaidic acid in HDL-PL has a negative effect on CUC.

In the present study, we found that the addition of rhLCAT to rHDL enhanced CUC, and LCAT-dependent enhancement of CUC was suppressed in rHDL containing elaidic acid in PC when compared to rHDL containing oleic acid, a cis analogue of elaidic acid. A previous study showed that the incorporation of structurally linear elaidic acid into PL reduces the fluidity of lipid membranes [19]. Therefore, elaidic acid could reduce the surface fluidity of HDL and attenuate CUC in the presence of LCAT. Additionally, the present study showed that LCAT was less reactive to PC containing elaidic acid than PC containing oleic acid, and affected the efficiency of cholesterol esterification in rHDL. A previous study showed that cholesterol esterification contributed to HDL maturation and increased the capacity of HDL to remove cholesterol [29,30]. Therefore, elaidic acid may affect the esterification of cholesterol in addition to membrane fluidity, thereby inhibiting cholesterol uptake and maturation of HDL. Although the mechanism by which elaidic acid affects LCAT reactivity has not been fully elucidated, considering that substrates of PL need to move into the active site of LCAT from HDL through the path that is made by the interaction between LCAT and apoA1 [42], elaidic acid may decrease the surface fluidity of HDL and reduce the efficiency of providing substrates of PL to LCAT through the path.

In this study, we did not perform a detailed structural analysis to elucidate how rHDL, which contains elaidic acid-PC, undergoes structural changes upon reaction with rhLCAT. Recently, the binding mode of LCAT and HDL was analyzed using negative stain electron microscopy (EM), validated with hydrogen–deuterium exchange mass spectrometry (HDX-MS) and crosslinking coupled with mass spectrometry (XL-MS) [42]. Adaptation of these techniques for rHDL analysis may reveal more detailed effects of elaidic acid-PC on LCAT-dependent HDL maturation in the future.

Recently, much attention has been focused on restoring or regulating HDL function to prevent atherosclerosis. Previously, we found that EPA enhanced CEC when it was incorporated into HDL [11,12]. In the present study, we found that elaidic acid incorporated in HDL-PL negatively affected CUC. In view of these results, modulation of the PL acyl groups may be an effective strategy to improve HDL function. CUC was significantly enhanced in the presence of rhLCAT. Recently, therapeutic concepts for coronary heart disease and atherosclerosis using recombinant LCAT protein or an LCAT activator have been proposed, and dose-dependent increases in HDL-C along with the enhancement of cholesterol efflux or in vivo reverse cholesterol transport (RCT) have been demonstrated [30,43]. Considering the enhancement of CUC in the presence of rhLCAT, as shown in this study, CUC may change in response to these molecules, in a manner similar to cholesterol efflux.

Study Limitations

This study has several limitations. First, because CUC is determined by a cell-free assay, CUC does not reflect the ABCA1 mediated cellular binding of apoA1 and the unidirectional export of cholesterol and PL to lipid-free/-poor apoA1 [7], which is considered as the first step of reverse cholesterol transport. Hence, the effect of elaidic acid in HDL-PL on cholesterol efflux remains to be elucidated. Second, we assessed rHDL containing only elaidic acid in PC for in vitro analysis. Since the concentrations of elaidic acid in vivo are much lower than those of other fatty acids, HDL containing such a highly enriched elaidic acid does not exist in vivo. However, considering the inverse association between CUC and the proportion of elaidic acid in HDL-PL observed in the correlation study using serum samples, we believe that our results reflect the intrinsic effect of elaidic acid on HDL. Further elucidation is required to address this issue. Third, although we used PC, which contains elaidic acid in both the sn1 and sn2 positions, as elaidic acid-PC, it is not consistent with a previous study that showed that PL contains saturated FA at position sn1 and unsaturated FA at position sn2 [35–37]. However, a previous study that assessed the membrane fluidity by steady-state fluorescence polarization of the probe diphenylhexatriene (DPH) showed that lipid membranes made from trans-containing PC (trans-PC) were less fluid than lipid membranes made from cis-containing PC (cis-PC), regardless of the position of incorporation (sn1 only, or both sn1 and sn2 of the glycerol backbone) [19]. Hence, we believe that the type of elaidic acid-PC used in our rHDL analysis did not affect the conclusions of this study. Fourth, we assessed rHDL containing the same amount of apoA1 for in vitro analysis. Since the interaction of LCAT to apoA1 enhances the enzymatic activity of LCAT [42], the amount of apoA1 per HDL particle and post-translational modifications of apoA1 such as nitration [44] may affect the LCAT-dependent cholesterol esterification and CUC. To address this issue, a comprehensive analysis using rHDL containing different amounts and qualities of apoA1 is needed.

Lastly, we did not assess the effects of polyunsaturated fatty acids, which may enhance lipid membrane fluidity. Further studies, such as comprehensive lipid profile assessment of HDL and analysis of rHDL composed of other types of phospholipids are needed to generalize the present findings.

5. Conclusions

The present study revealed that CUC is affected by the HDL-PL level. Moreover, CUC was negatively associated with the proportion of elaidic acid in HDL-PL, suggesting that the composition of HDL-PL is also a determinant factor of CUC. In vitro analysis using rHDL showed that CUC was positively affected by LCAT-dependent cholesterol esterification, whereas the incorporation of elaidic acid in HDL-PL attenuated the cholesterol esterification efficiency by LCAT in addition to decreasing the fluidity of the HDL surface as reported previously, thereby inhibiting the process of cholesterol uptake and maturation of HDL. Further analysis to elucidate the regulatory mechanisms of CUC will lead to new diagnostic and therapeutic strategies for atherosclerosis and cardiovascular disease.

Supplementary Materials: The following are available online at https://www.mdpi.com/article/10.3390/nu13093112/s1, Figure S1: Correlations between CUC and elaidic acid or oleic acid in HDL-PL; Table S1: Detailed laboratory data; Table S2: Detailed baseline patient characteristics.

Author Contributions: Conceptualization, T.I. (Takuya Iino), R.T., M.N. (Manabu Nagao), Y.I.; methodology, T.I. (Takuya Iino), M.S., A.H. and K.M., Y.I.; software, T.I. (Takuya Iino) and M.S.; validation, T.I. (Takuya Iino), R.T., M.N. (Manabu Nagao), M.S., Y.I., M.N. (Makoto Nishimori), S.Y., Y.S., T.I. (Tatsuro Ishida), and K.-i.H.; formal analysis, T.I. (Takuya Iino); investigation, T.I. (Takuya

Iino); resources, M.S.; data curation, T.I. (Takuya Iino); writing—original draft preparation, T.I. (Takuya Iino); writing—review and editing, R.T., M.N. (Manabu Nagao); visualization, T.I. (Takuya Iino); supervision, R.T., T.I. (Tatsuro Ishida) and K.-i.H.; project administration, R.T., T.I. (Tatsuro Ishida) and K.-i.H.; funding acquisition, R.T., Y.I., T.I. (Tatsuro Ishida) and K.-i.H. All authors have read and agreed to the published version of the manuscript.

Funding: Institutional funding by Sysmex Corporation and Grant-in-Aid for Scientific Research (C) 19K08490 and 20K17081 from the Ministry of Education, Culture, Sports, Science and Technology of Japan.

Institutional Review Board Statement: The study protocol was in accordance with the ethical guidelines of the 1975 Declaration of Helsinki. The study was approved by the Ethics Review Committee at Kobe University (Japan) and was registered in the UMIN Clinical Trials Registry (identification number 000030297).

Informed Consent Statement: Informed consent was obtained from all subjects involved in the study.

Data Availability Statement: Not applicable.

Conflicts of Interest: The Division of Evidence-based Laboratory Medicine, Kobe University Graduate School of Medicine, was established by an endowment fund from the Sysmex Corporation. Takuya Iino, Amane Harada, Katsuhiro Murakami, Yasuhiro Irino are employees of the Sysmex Corporation.

Appendix A. Supplemental Methods

Appendix A.1. Generation of Mouse Monoclonal Antibody 8E10 and P1A5

Hybridoma cell lines were generated by immunizing C57BL/6 mice with recombinant human apoA1 protein (Merck KGaA, Darmstadt, Germany). Mouse immunization and generation of hybridoma cell lines were outsourced to the Cell Engineering Corporation (Osaka, Japan). Hybridoma culture supernatants containing antibodies with the desired binding specificity for equal recognition of non-oxidized and oxidized HDL were screened by ELISA. In brief, 1 µg/mL of recombinant human apoA1 protein or apoB-depleted serum with an apoA1 concentration of 1 µg/mL, diluted in PBS, were immobilized on 96-well plates at 37 °C for 1 h. After washing the wells with PBS, PBS with or without hydrogen peroxide (H_2O_2), sodium nitrite, and diethylenetriaminepentaacetic acid (DTPA) solution (final concentrations of 1 mol/L, 200 µmol/L, and 100 µmol/L, respectively) were added to the wells and incubated at 37 °C for 1 h. The wells were washed with PBS and blocked with 2% BSA in PBS at 25 °C for 1 h. The plates were then incubated with hybridoma culture supernatant at 25 °C for 1 h, followed by the addition of horseradish peroxidase (HRP)-conjugated goat anti-mouse IgG (Dako, Glostrup, Denmark) at 25 °C for 30 min. The wells were washed with PBS five times, SuperSignal ELISA pico chemiluminescent substrate (Thermo Fisher Scientific, Inc., Waltham, MA, USA) was added to the wells, and the chemiluminescence signal was measured using an Infinite F200 Pro microplate reader (Tecan, Mannedorf, Switzerland). The mAb 8E10 and P1A5 were selected by screening for equal recognition of lipid-free (recombinant protein) and lipidated (apoB-depleted serum) apoA1 under native conditions, as well as after oxidation by exposure to H_2O_2/NO_2^-. In order to obtain sufficient antibodies for this study, mAb 8E10 was purified from the ascites fluid of ICR nude mice by Protein A-Sepharose chromatography. Preparation of mouse ascites fluid and purification of mAb 8E10 and P1A5 were outsourced to Kitayama Labs (Nagano, Japan).

Appendix A.2. Synthesis of Biotin-PEG7-Cholesterol

Fifteen milligrams of 3β-Hydroxy-Δ^5-cholenic Acid (Wako) were dissolved in 500 µL of N,N-dimethylformamide. Then, 7.7 mg of 1-Ethyl-3-(3-dimethylaminopropyl) carbodiimide, hydrochloride (Dojindo), 4.6 mg of N-hydroxysuccinimide (Merck KGaA, Darmstadt, Germany), 23.8 mg of Biotin-PEG7-amine (BroadPharm), and 8.4 µL of triethylamine (Wako) were added, and the resulting solution was stirred at room temperature for 2 h.

Silica gel column chromatography (10% methanol in chloroform) yielded Biotin-PEG7-cholesterol as a clear solid (4% yield). LC-MS (*m/z*): 951.4 [M + H]$^+$.

References

1. Khera, A.V.; Cuchel, M.; De La Llera-Moya, M.; Rodrigues, A.; Burke, M.F.; Jafri, K.; French, B.C.; Phillips, J.A.; Mucksavage, M.L.; Wilensky, R.L.; et al. Cholesterol Efflux Capacity, High-Density Lipoprotein Function, and Atherosclerosis. *N. Engl. J. Med.* **2011**, *364*, 127–135. [CrossRef]
2. Rohatgi, A.; Khera, A.; Berry, J.D.; Givens, E.G.; Ayers, C.R.; Wedin, K.E.; Neeland, I.J.; Yuhanna, I.S.; Rader, D.R.; De Lemos, J.A.; et al. HDL Cholesterol Efflux Capacity and Incident Cardiovascular Events. *N. Engl. J. Med.* **2014**, *371*, 2383–2393. [CrossRef]
3. Saleheen, D.; Scott, R.; Javad, S.; Zhao, W.; Rodrigues, A.; Picataggi, A.; Lukmanova, D.; Mucksavage, M.L.; Luben, R.; Billheimer, J.; et al. Association of HDL cholesterol efflux capacity with incident coronary heart disease events: A prospective case-control study. *Lancet Diabetes Endocrinol.* **2015**, *3*, 507–513. [CrossRef]
4. Anastasius, M.; Kockx, M.; Jessup, W.; Sullivan, D.; Rye, K.-A.; Kritharides, L. Cholesterol efflux capacity: An introduction for clinicians. *Am. Heart J.* **2016**, *180*, 54–63. [CrossRef]
5. Rothblat, G.H.; de la Llera-Moya, M.; Atger, V.; Kellner-Weibel, G.; Williams, D.L.; Phillips, M.C. Cell cholesterol efflux: Integration of old and new observations provides new insights. *J. Lipid Res.* **1999**, *40*, 781–796. [CrossRef]
6. Harada, A.; Toh, R.; Murakami, K.; Kiriyama, M.; Yoshikawa, K.; Miwa, K.; Kubo, T.; Irino, Y.; Mori, K.; Tanaka, N.; et al. Cholesterol Uptake Capacity: A New Measure of HDL Functionality for Coronary Risk Assessment. *J. Appl. Lab. Med.* **2017**, *2*, 186–200. [CrossRef]
7. Toh, R. Assessment of HDL Cholesterol Removal Capacity: Toward Clinical Application. *J. Atheroscler. Thromb.* **2019**, *26*, 111–120. [CrossRef]
8. Agnani, G.; Marcel, Y.L. Cholesterol efflux from fibroblasts to discoidal lipoproteins with apolipoprotein A-I (LpA-I) increases with particle size but cholesterol transfer from LpA-I to lipoproteins decreases with size. *Biochemistry* **1993**, *32*, 2643–2649. [CrossRef]
9. Davidson, W.S.; Lund-Katz, S.; Johnson, W.J.; Anantharamaiah, G.M.; Palgunachari, M.N.; Segrest, J.P.; Rothblat, G.H.; Phil-lips, M.C. The Influence of Apolipoprotein Structure on the Efflux of Cellular Free Cholesterol to High Density Lipopro-tein. *J. Biol. Chem.* **1994**, *269*, 22975–22982. [CrossRef]
10. Davidson, W.; Gillotte, K.L.; Lund-Katz, S.; Johnson, W.J.; Rothblat, G.H.; Phillips, M.C. The Effect of High Density Lipoprotein Phospholipid Acyl Chain Composition on the Efflux of Cellular Free Cholesterol. *J. Biol. Chem.* **1995**, *270*, 5882–5890. [CrossRef] [PubMed]
11. Tanaka, N.; Ishida, T.; Nagao, M.; Mori, T.; Monguchi, T.; Sasaki, M.; Mori, K.; Kondo, K.; Nakajima, H.; Honjo, T.; et al. Administration of high dose eicosapentaenoic acid enhances anti-inflammatory properties of high-density lipoprotein in Japanese patients with dyslipidemia. *Atherosclerosis* **2014**, *237*, 577–583. [CrossRef]
12. Tanaka, N.; Irino, Y.; Shinohara, M.; Tsuda, S.; Mori, T.; Nagao, M.; Oshita, T.; Mori, K.; Hara, T.; Toh, R.; et al. Eicosapentaenoic Acid-Enriched High-Density Lipoproteins Exhibit Anti-Atherogenic Properties. *Circ. J.* **2018**, *82*, 596–601. [CrossRef]
13. Mori, K.; Ishida, T.; Yasuda, T.; Hasokawa, M.; Monguchi, T.; Sasaki, M.; Mori, K.; Nakajima, H.; Shinohara, M.; Shinke, T.; et al. Serum Trans-Fatty Acid Concentration Is Elevated in Young Patients With Coronary Artery Disease in Japan. *Circ. J.* **2015**, *79*, 2017–2025. [CrossRef]
14. Oshita, T.; Toh, R.; Shinohara, M.; Mori, K.; Irino, Y.; Nagao, M.; Hara, T.; Otake, H.; Ishida, T.; Hirata, K.-I. Elevated Serum Elaidic Acid Predicts Risk of Repeat Revascularization After Percutaneous Coronary Intervention in Japan. *Circ. J.* **2019**, *83*, 1032–1038. [CrossRef]
15. Mozaffarian, D.; Aro, A.; Willett, W.C. Health effects of trans-fatty acids: Experimental and observational evidence. *Eur. J. Clin. Nutr.* **2009**, *63*, S5–S21. [CrossRef]
16. Willett, W.; Stampfer, M.; Manson, J.; Colditz, G.; Speizer, F.; Rosner, B.; Hennekens, C.; Sampson, L. Intake of trans fatty acids and risk of coronary heart disease among women. *Lancet* **1993**, *341*, 581–585. [CrossRef]
17. Mozaffarian, D.; Katan, M.B.; Ascherio, A.; Stampfer, M.J.; Willett, W.C. Trans Fatty Acids and Cardiovascular Disease. *N. Engl. J. Med.* **2006**, *354*, 1601–1613. [CrossRef]
18. Vidgren, H.M.; Louheranta, A.M.; Ågren, J.J.; Schwab, U.S.; Uusitupa, M.I.J. Divergent incorporation of dietary trans fatty acids in different serum lipid fractions. *Lipids* **1998**, *33*, 955–962. [CrossRef] [PubMed]
19. Roach, C.; Feller, S.E.; Ward, J.A.; Shaikh, S.R.; Zerouga, M.; Stillwell, W. Comparison of Cis and Trans Fatty Acid Containing Phosphatidylcholines on Membrane Properties†. *Biochemistry* **2004**, *43*, 6344–6351. [CrossRef]
20. Kontush, A.; Lhomme, M.; Chapman, M.J. Unraveling the complexities of the HDL lipidome. *J. Lipid Res.* **2013**, *54*, 2950–2963. [CrossRef]
21. Davidson, W.; Heink, A.; Sexmith, H.; Melchior, J.T.; Gordon, S.M.; Kuklenyik, Z.; Woollett, L.; Barr, J.R.; Jones, J.; Toth, C.; et al. The effects of apolipoprotein B depletion on HDL subspecies composition and function. *J. Lipid Res.* **2016**, *57*, 674–686. [CrossRef]
22. Bligh, E.G.; Dyer, W.J. A rapid method of total lipid extraction and purification. *Can. J. Biochem. Physiol.* **1959**, *37*, 911–917. [CrossRef]
23. Cavigiolio, G.; Shao, B.; Geier, E.G.; Ren, G.; Heinecke, J.W.; Oda, M.N. The Interplay between Size, Morphology, Stability, and Functionality of High-Density Lipoprotein Subclasses. *Biochemistry* **2008**, *47*, 4770–4779. [CrossRef]

24. Sakurai, T.; Sakurai, A.; Vaisman, B.L.; Nishida, T.; Neufeld, E.B.; Demosky, S.J.; Sampson, M.L.; Shamburek, R.D.; Freeman, L.A.; Remaley, A.T. Development of a novel fluorescent activity assay for lecithin:cholesterol acyltransferase. *Ann. Clin. Biochem.* **2017**, *55*, 414–421. [CrossRef]
25. Teramoto, T.; Sasaki, J.; Ishibashi, S.; Birou, S.; Daida, H.; Dohi, S.; Egusa, G.; Hiro, T.; Hirobe, K.; Iida, M.; et al. Diagnosis of Atherosclerosis. Executive Summary of the Japan Atherosclerosis Society (JAS) Guidelines for the Diagnosis and Prevention of Atherosclerotic Cardiovascular Diseases in Japan—2012 Version. *J. Atheroscler. Thromb.* **2014**, *21*, 296–298. [CrossRef]
26. Rousset, X.; Vaisman, B.; Amar, M.; Sethi, A.A.; Remaley, A.T. Lecithin: Cholesterol acyltransferase—From biochemistry to role in cardiovascular disease. *Curr. Opin. Endocrinol. Diabetes Obes.* **2009**, *16*, 163–171. [CrossRef]
27. Schaefer, E.J.; Anthanont, P.; Asztalos, B.F. High-density lipoprotein metabolism, composition, function, and deficiency. *Curr. Opin. Lipidol.* **2014**, *25*, 194–199. [CrossRef]
28. Sorci-Thomas, M.G.; Bhat, S.; Thomas, M.J. Activation of lecithin:cholesterol acyltransferase by HDL ApoA-I central helices. *Clin. Lipidol.* **2009**, *4*, 113–124. [CrossRef]
29. Czarnecka, H.; Yokoyama, S. Regulation of Cellular Cholesterol Efflux by Lecithin:Cholesterol Acyltransferase Reaction through Nonspecific Lipid Exchange. *J. Biol. Chem.* **1996**, *271*, 2023–2028. [CrossRef]
30. Shamburek, R.D.; Bakker-Arkema, R.; Shamburek, A.M.; Freeman, L.A.; Amar, M.J.; Auerbach, B.; Krause, B.R.; Homan, R.; Adelman, S.J.; Collins, H.L.; et al. Safety and Tolerability of ACP-501, a Recombinant Human Lecithin:Cholesterol Acyltransferase, in a Phase 1 Single-Dose Escalation Study. *Circ. Res.* **2016**, *118*, 73–82. [CrossRef] [PubMed]
31. Khovidhunkit, W.; Shigenaga, J.K.; Moser, A.H.; Feingold, K.R.; Grunfeld, C. Cholesterol Efflux by Acute-Phase High Den-sity Lipoprotein: Role of Lecithin: Cholesterol Acyltransferase. *J. Lipid Res.* **2001**, *42*, 967–975. [CrossRef]
32. Stein, O.; Goren, R.; Stein, Y. Removal of cholesterol from fibroblasts and smooth muscle cells in culture in the presence and absence of cholesterol esterification in the medium. *Biochim. Biophys. Acta (BBA)-Lipids Lipid Metab.* **1978**, *529*, 309–318. [CrossRef]
33. Ray, E.; Bellini, F.; Stoudt, G.; Hemperly, S.; Rothblat, G. Influence of lecithin:cholesterol acyltransferase on cholesterol metabolism in hepatoma cells and hepatocytes. *Biochim. Biophys. Acta (BBA)-Lipids Lipid Metab.* **1980**, *617*, 318–334. [CrossRef]
34. Czarnecka, H.; Yokoyama, S. Lecithin:cholesterol acyltransferase reaction on cellular lipid released by free apolipoprotein-mediated efflux. *Biochemistry* **1995**, *34*, 4385–4392. [CrossRef]
35. Lands, W.E.; Merkl, I. Metabolism of Glycerolipids. III. Reactivity of Various Acyl Esters of Coenzyme A With Al-pha′-Acylglycerophosphorylcholine, and Positional Specificities in Lecithin Synthesis. *J. Biol. Chem.* **1963**, *238*, 898–904. [CrossRef]
36. Yabuuchi, H.; O'Brien, J.S. Positional distribution of fatty acids in glycerophosphatides of bovine gray matter. *J. Lipid Res.* **1968**, *9*, 65–67. [CrossRef]
37. Manni, M.M.; Tiberti, M.L.; Pagnotta, S.; Barelli, H.; Gautier, R.; Antonny, B. Acyl chain asymmetry and polyunsaturation of brain phospholipids facilitate membrane vesiculation without leakage. *eLife* **2018**, *7*, e34394. [CrossRef] [PubMed]
38. Fournier, N.; Paul, J.-L.; Atger, V.; Cogny, A.; Soni, T.; de la Llera-Moya, M.; Rothblat, G.; Moatti, N. HDL Phospholipid Content and Composition as a Major Factor Determining Cholesterol Efflux Capacity From Fu5AH Cells to Human Serum. *Arter. Thromb. Vasc. Biol.* **1997**, *17*, 2685–2691. [CrossRef]
39. Sankaranarayanan, S.; Oram, J.F.; Asztalos, B.F.; Vaughan, A.M.; Lund-Katz, S.; Adorni, M.P.; Phillips, M.C.; Rothblat, G.H. Effects of acceptor composition and mechanism of ABCG1-mediated cellular free cholesterol efflux. *J. Lipid Res.* **2009**, *50*, 275–284. [CrossRef]
40. Berg, J.M.; Tymoczko, J.L.; Stryer, L. There Are Three Common Types of Membrane Lipids. In *Biochemistry*, 5th ed.; WH Freeman: New York, NY, USA, 2002; Volume 5.
41. Hunter, J.E. Dietary trans fatty acids: Review of recent human studies and food industry responses. *Lipids* **2006**, *41*, 967–992. [CrossRef]
42. Manthei, K.A.; Patra, D.; Wilson, C.J.; Fawaz, M.V.; Piersimoni, L.; Shenkar, J.C.; Yuan, W.; Andrews, P.; Engen, J.R.; Schwendeman, A.; et al. Structural analysis of lecithin:cholesterol acyltransferase bound to high density lipoprotein particles. *Commun. Biol.* **2020**, *3*, 28. [CrossRef]
43. Sasaki, M.; Delaware, M.; Sakurai, H.; Kobayashi, H.; Nakao, N.; Tsuru, H.; Fukushima, Y.; Honzumi, S.; Moriyama, S.; Wada, N.; et al. Novel LCAT (Lecithin:Cholesterol Acyltransferase) Activator DS-8190a Prevents the Progression of Plaque Accumulation in Atherosclerosis Models. *Arter. Thromb. Vasc. Biol.* **2020**, *41*, 360–376. [CrossRef] [PubMed]
44. DiDonato, J.A.; Aulak, K.; Huang, Y.; Wagner, M.; Gerstenecker, G.; Topbas, C.; Gogonea, V.; DiDonato, A.J.; Tang, W.H.W.; Mehl, R.A.; et al. Site-specific Nitration of Apolipoprotein A-I at Tyrosine 166 Is Both Abundant within Human Atherosclerotic Plaque and Dysfunctional. *J. Biol. Chem.* **2014**, *289*, 10276–10292. [CrossRef] [PubMed]

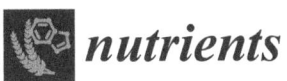

Article

Association of Body Mass Index with Ischemic and Hemorrhagic Stroke

Masahiro Shiozawa [1], Hidehiro Kaneko [1,2,*], Hidetaka Itoh [1], Kojiro Morita [3], Akira Okada [4], Satoshi Matsuoka [1,5], Hiroyuki Kiriyama [1], Tatsuya Kamon [1], Katsuhito Fujiu [1,2], Nobuaki Michihata [6], Taisuke Jo [6], Norifumi Takeda [1], Hiroyuki Morita [1], Sunao Nakamura [5], Koichi Node [7], Hideo Yasunaga [8] and Issei Komuro [1]

1. The Department of Cardiovascular Medicine, The University of Tokyo, Tokyo 113-8655, Japan; m.palesaxeblue3205@gmail.com (M.S.); hitoh.ggl@gmail.com (H.I.); s-matsuoka@shin-tokyohospital.or.jp (S.M.); kiriyaman0427@gmail.com (H.K.); kamont-int@h.u-tokyo.ac.jp (T.K.); fujiu-tky@g.ecc.u-tokyo.ac.jp (K.F.); norifutakeda@gmail.com (N.T.); hiroymorita@gmail.com (H.M.); komuro_tky2000@yahoo.co.jp (I.K.)
2. The Department of Advanced Cardiology, The University of Tokyo, Tokyo 113-8655, Japan
3. Global Nursing Research Center, Graduate School of Medicine, The University of Tokyo, Tokyo 113-8655, Japan; kojiromorita7@gmail.com
4. Department of Prevention of Diabetes and Lifestyle-Related Diseases, Graduate School of Medicine, The University of Tokyo, Tokyo 113-8655, Japan; aokada@m.u-tokyo.ac.jp
5. The Department of Cardiology, New Tokyo Hospital, Matsudo 270-2232, Japan; boss0606@pluto.plala.or.jp
6. The Department of Health Services Research, The University of Tokyo, Tokyo 113-0033, Japan; gha10771@gmail.com (N.M.); jo.taisuke@gmail.com (T.J.)
7. Department of Cardiovascular Medicine, Saga University, Saga 849-8501, Japan; node@cc.saga-u.ac.jp
8. The Department of Clinical Epidemiology and Health Economics, School of Public Health, The University of Tokyo, Tokyo 113-0033, Japan; yasunagah@m.u-tokyo.ac.jp
* Correspondence: hidehikaneko-circ@umin.ac.jp or kanekohidehiro@gmail.com; Tel.: +81-33815-5411; Fax: +81-35800-9171

Abstract: Data on the association between body mass index (BMI) and stroke are scarce. We aimed to examine the association between BMI and incident stroke (ischemic or hemorrhagic) and to clarify the relationship between underweight, overweight, and obesity and stroke risk stratified by sex. We analyzed the JMDC Claims Database between January 2005 and April 2020 including 2,740,778 healthy individuals (Median (interquartile) age, 45 (38–53) years; 56.2% men; median (interquartile) BMI, 22.3 (20.2–24.8) kg/m^2). None of the participants had a history of cardiovascular disease. Each participant was categorized as underweight (BMI <18.5 kg/m^2), normal weight (BMI 18.5–24.9 kg/m^2), overweight (BMI 25.0–29.9 kg/m^2), or obese (BMI ≥ 30 kg/m^2). We investigated the association of BMI with incidence stroke in men and women using the Cox regression model. We used restricted cubic spline (RCS) functions to identify the association of BMI as a continuous parameter with incident stroke. The incidence (95% confidence interval) of total stroke, ischemic stroke, and hemorrhagic stroke was 32.5 (32.0–32.9), 28.1 (27.6–28.5), and 5.5 (5.3–5.7) per 10,000 person-years in men, whereas 25.7 (25.1–26.2), 22.5 (22.0–23.0), and 4.0 (3.8–4.2) per 10,000 person-years in women, respectively. Multivariable Cox regression analysis showed that overweight and obesity were associated with a higher incidence of total and ischemic stroke in both men and women. Underweight, overweight, and obesity were associated with a higher hemorrhagic stroke incidence in men, but not in women. Restricted cubic spline showed that the risk of ischemic stroke increased in a BMI dose-dependent manner in both men and women, whereas there was a U-shaped relationship between BMI and the hemorrhagic stroke risk in men. In conclusion, overweight and obesity were associated with a greater incidence of stroke and ischemic stroke in both men and women. Furthermore, underweight, overweight, and obesity were associated with a higher hemorrhagic stroke risk in men. Our results would help in the risk stratification of future stroke based on BMI.

Keywords: body mass index; obesity; underweight; ischemic stroke; hemorrhagic stroke

Citation: Shiozawa, M.; Kaneko, H.; Itoh, H.; Morita, K.; Okada, A.; Matsuoka, S.; Kiriyama, H.; Kamon, T.; Fujiu, K.; Michihata, N.; et al. Association of Body Mass Index with Ischemic and Hemorrhagic Stroke. *Nutrients* 2021, 13, 2343. https://doi.org/10.3390/nu13072343

Academic Editor: Hayato Tada

Received: 13 June 2021
Accepted: 29 June 2021
Published: 9 July 2021

Publisher's Note: MDPI stays neutral with regard to jurisdictional claims in published maps and institutional affiliations.

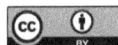

Copyright: © 2021 by the authors. Licensee MDPI, Basel, Switzerland. This article is an open access article distributed under the terms and conditions of the Creative Commons Attribution (CC BY) license (https://creativecommons.org/licenses/by/4.0/).

1. Introduction

Stroke is a major cause of death and disability [1–3]. In the United States, the annual incidence of stroke is approximately 795,000, of which approximately 610,000 are first-ever stroke events, and 185,000 are recurrent stroke events [1]. In the European countries, there were 2.3 million new cases diagnosed with stroke and 20.4 million people living with stroke in 2017 [4]. Obesity is an important risk factor for cardiovascular disease (CVD) [5–9] and is reported to be associated with a greater incidence of stroke [10–12]. Conversely, underweight is also associated with a higher risk of several CVDs and adverse clinical outcomes [13–15]. However, the data on the risk of underweight with incident stroke are scarce. Moreover, stroke can be categorized into two types, ischemic stroke, and hemorrhagic stroke; additionally, the pathology of these two subtypes should be separately discussed. For example, several studies have shown that body mass index (BMI) could influence the risk of ischemic or hemorrhagic stroke differently [16,17]. However, the association of wide-range BMI (including both obesity and underweight) with incident ischemic or hemorrhagic stroke has not been fully elucidated [10–12,16,17]. Furthermore, the distribution of BMI is different between men and women; therefore, the relationship between BMI and the risk of stroke could differ by sex [10,12]. In this study, we sought to examine the relationship between BMI and incident ischemic or hemorrhagic stroke stratified by sex using a nationwide epidemiological database.

2. Methods

The data from the JMDC Claims Database are available for anyone who would purchase it from JMDC Inc. (JMDC Inc.; Tokyo, Japan), which is a healthcare venture company in Tokyo, Japan.

2.1. Study Population

We conducted this retrospective observational study using the JMDC Claims Database between January 2005 and April 2020 [18–23]. The JMDC Claims Database includes the health insurance claims data from more than 60 insurers. The majority of insured individuals enrolled in the JMDC Claims Database are employees of relatively large companies. The JMDC Claims Database includes the individuals' health check-up data, including demographics, prior medical history, medication status, and hospital claims recorded using the International Classification of Diseases, 10th Revision (ICD-10) coding. JMDC which is a healthcare venture company, collected the data on health check-up and clinical outcome such as diagnosis of stroke using ICD-10 code from insurer or medical institutes regularly, and assembled a database. We extracted 3,621,942 individuals with available health check-up data on BMI (12.5–60 kg/m^2), blood pressure, and blood test results at health check-up from the JMDC Claims Database between January 2005 and April 2020. Subsequently, we excluded the individuals with a history of myocardial infarction, angina pectoris, stroke, heart failure, and atrial fibrillation or hemodialysis (n = 166,144), and those with missing data on medications for hypertension, diabetes mellitus, or dyslipidemia (n = 222,496), cigarette smoking (n = 15,404), alcohol consumption (n = 370,041), and physical inactivity (n = 107,079). Finally, 2,740,778 participants were included in this study (Figure 1).

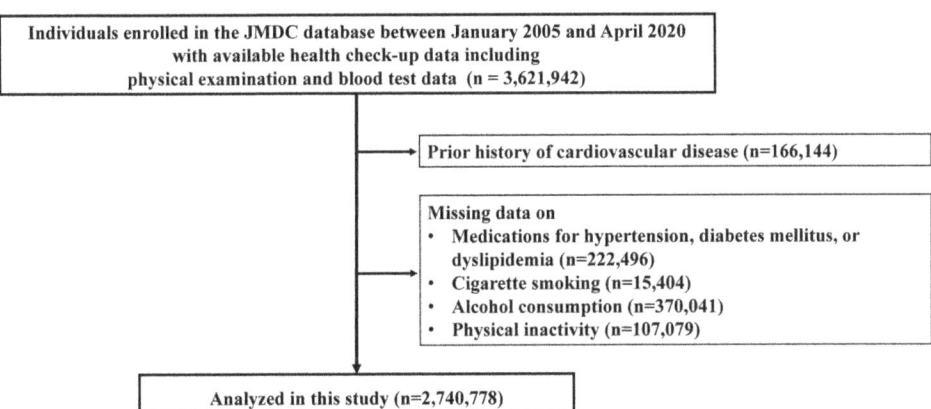

Figure 1. Flowchart. We extracted 3,621,942 individuals with available health check-up data including physical examination and blood test from the JMDC Claims Database between January 2005 and April 2020. We excluded individuals with CVD history of myocardial infarction, angina pectoris, stroke, heart failure, and atrial fibrillation or hemodialysis (n = 166,144), and those having missing data on medications for hypertension, diabetes mellitus, or dyslipidemia (n = 222,496), cigarette smoking (n = 15,404), alcohol consumption (n = 370,041), and physical inactivity (n = 107,079). Finally, we included 2,740,778 participants in this study.

2.2. Ethics

This study was conducted according to the ethical guidelines of our institution (approval by the Ethical Committee of The University of Tokyo: 2018–10862) and in accordance with the principles of the Declaration of Helsinki. The requirement for informed consent was waived because all the data from the JMDC Claims Database were de-identified.

2.3. Category of Body Mass Index

We categorized the study participants into four groups: underweight, normal weight, overweight, and obesity defined as BMI <18.5 kg/m^2, 18.5–24.9 kg/m^2, 25.0–29.9 kg/m^2 and $\geq$30 kg/m^2, respectively [14].

2.4. Measurements and Definitions

The data, including BMI, history of hypertension, diabetes mellitus, dyslipidemia, CVD, blood pressure, and fasting laboratory values were collected using standardized protocols at the health check-up. The information on cigarette smoking (current or non-current) and alcohol consumption (every day or not every day) were self-reported. Hypertension was defined as systolic blood pressure $\geq$ 140 mmHg, diastolic blood pressure $\geq$ 90 mmHg, or the use of blood pressure-lowering medications. Diabetes mellitus was defined as fasting glucose level $\geq$ 126 mg/dL or the use of glucose-lowering medications. Dyslipidemia was defined as low-density lipoprotein cholesterol level $\geq$ 140 mg/dL, high-density lipoprotein cholesterol level <40 mg/dL, triglyceride level $\geq$ 150 mg/dL, or the use of lipid-lowering medications. Physical inactivity was defined as not engaging in at least 30 min of exercise two or more times a week or not walking $\geq$ 1 h per day, as previously described [24].

2.5. Outcomes

The outcomes were collected between January 2005 and April 2020. The primary outcome was stroke (ICD-10: I630, I631, I632, I633, I634, I635, I636, I638, I639, I600, I601, I602, I603, I604, I605, I606, I607, I608, I609, I610, I611, I613, I614, I615, I616, I619, I629, and G459). We defined ischemic stroke as I630, I631, I632, I633, I634, I635, I636, I638, I639, and G459, and hemorrhagic stroke as I600, I601, I602, I603, I604, I605. I606, I607, I608, I609, I610, I611, I613, I614, I615, I616, I619, and I629.

2.6. Statistical Analysis

We analyzed the study population stratified by sex. The data are expressed as median (interquartile range) for continuous variables or number (percentage) for categorical variables. The summary statistics for the characteristics of participants between the four categories based on BMI were calculated. The statistical significance of differences among the four categories was determined using analysis of variance for continuous variables and chi-squared tests for categorical variables. We conducted Cox regression analyses to identify the association between BMI categories and incident stroke. The hazard ratios (HRs) were calculated in an unadjusted model (Model 1), an age-adjusted model (Model 2), and after adjustment for age, hypertension, diabetes mellitus, dyslipidemia, cigarette smoking, alcohol consumption, and physical inactivity (Model 3). We performed three sensitivity analyses. First, we analyzed the relationship between BMI as a continuous variable and incident stroke. To detect any possible linear or non-linear dependency in regression models and to allow for a flexible interpretation of the relationship between BMI as continuous data and stroke events, continuous changes in BMI were assessed through shape-restricted cubic spline (RCS) regression models. We put three cut-off points for BMI (18.5, 25.0, and 30.0 kg/m^2) as the knots. HRs and 95% confidence interval (CI) for incident stroke were calculated for each value of BMI with respect to the reference BMI value of 23.0 kg/m^2. Second, we used multiple imputation for missing data, as previously described. [18,25] On the assumption of data missing at random, we imputed the missing data for covariates using the chained equation method with 20 iterations as described by Aloisio [26]. The HRs and standard errors were obtained using Rubin's rules [27]. Third, we analyzed the population after excluding hypertensive participants. The statistical significance was set at $p < 0.05$. The statistical analyses were performed using SPSS software (version 25, SPSS Inc., Chicago, IL, USA) and STATA (version 17; StataCorp LLC, College Station, TX, USA).

3. Results

3.1. Baseline Clinical Characteristics

The baseline clinical characteristics are shown in Table 1. Overall, the median (interquartile range) age was 45 (38–53) years, and 1,538,982 participants (56.2%) were men. The median (interquartile range) BMI was 23.2 (21.3–25.5) kg/m^2 in men and 21.0 (19.2–23.4) kg/m^2 in women. The prevalence of hypertension, diabetes mellitus, and dyslipidemia increased with BMI in both men and women.

Table 1. Clinical Characteristics of Study Population.

	Men					Women				
	Body Mass Index Category					Body Mass Index Category				
	Normal-Weight (n = 1,013,302)	Under-Weight (n = 61,704)	Over-Weight (n = 382,425)	Obesity (n = 81,551)	p-Value	Normal-Weight (n = 832,491)	Under-Weight (n = 180,421)	Over-Weight (n = 146,243)	Obesity (n = 42,641)	p-Value
Body Mass Index, kg/m^2	22.2 (20.9–23.5)	17.7 (17.1–18.1)	26.5 (25.7–27.8)	31.9 (30.8–33.9)	<0.001	21.0 (19.7–22.5)	17.7 (17.0–18.1)	26.6 (25.7–27.9)	32.2 (30.9–34.4)	<0.001
Age	45 (38–53)	40 (28–49)	46 (40–54)	44 (38–50)	<0.001	44 (38–52)	42 (35–50)	47 (41–55)	45 (40–52)	<0.001
Hypertension	168,808 (16.7)	4403 (7.1)	125,180 (32.7)	40,933 (50.2)	<0.001	78,824 (9.5)	8078 (4.5)	36,944 (25.3)	17,570 (41.2)	<0.001
Diabetes Mellitus	38,041 (3.8)	1321 (2.1)	34,687 (9.1)	15,508 (19.0)	<0.001	10,050 (1.2)	984 (0.5)	8101 (5.5)	5345 (12.5)	<0.001
Dyslipidemia	402,085 (39.7)	8569 (13.9)	249,118 (65.1)	59,961 (73.5)	<0.001	218,254 (26.2)	24,740 (13.7)	73,805 (50.5)	25,321 (59.4)	<0.001
Cigarette Smoking	358,087 (35.3)	26,057 (42.2)	138,997 (36.3)	30,566 (37.5)	<0.001	89,573 (10.8)	21,531 (11.9)	18,698 (12.8)	6501 (15.2)	<0.001
Alcohol Drinking	334,709 (33.0)	15,635 (25.3)	111,393 (29.1)	13,905 (17.1)	<0.001	106,545 (12.8)	21,594 (12.0)	14,257 (9.7)	2680 (6.3)	<0.001
Physical Inactivity	511,731 (50.5)	31,675 (51.3)	208,506 (54.5)	47,022 (57.7)	<0.001	438,299 (52.6)	96,282 (53.4)	82,529 (56.4)	25,767 (60.4)	<0.001

Table 1. Cont.

	Men					Women				
	Body Mass Index Category					Body Mass Index Category				
	Normal-Weight (n = 1,013,302)	Under-Weight (n = 61,704)	Over-Weight (n = 382,425)	Obesity (n = 81,551)	p-Value	Normal-Weight (n = 832,491)	Under-Weight (n = 180,421)	Over-Weight (n = 146,243)	Obesity (n = 42,641)	p-Value
SBP, mmHg	119 (110–128)	112 (104–122)	126 (117–135)	131 (123–141)	<0.001	111 (102–122)	106 (98–116)	122 (112–133)	129 (120–140)	<0.001
DBP, mmHg	74 (67–81)	69 (62–76)	80 (72–86)	83 (76–90)	<0.001	68 (61–76)	65 (59–72)	75 (68–83)	80 (72–88)	<0.001
Glucose, mg/dL	92 (87–99)	89 (84–95)	96 (89–105)	99 (91–113)	<0.001	89 (84–94)	86 (82–92)	93 (87–100)	97 (90–107)	<0.001
LDL-C/mg/dL	119 (99–140)	98 (82–117)	130 (110–151)	132 (112–153)	<0.001	113 (94–135)	102 (86–122)	129 (108–151)	132 (113–154)	<0.001
HDL-C, mg/dL	59 (50–69)	66 (57–77)	51 (44–59)	47 (41–54)	<0.001	71 (61–81)	76 (67–87)	61 (52–71)	55 (48–64)	<0.001
Triglycerides, mg/dL	88 (63–127)	64 (48–85)	125 (88–181)	141 (101–202)	<0.001	63 (48–87)	55 (43–71)	91 (66–128)	107 (79–149)	<0.001

Data are reported as medians (interquartile range) and proportions (percentage). p values were calculated using chi-square tests for categorical variables and the analysis of variance for continuous variables. Participants were categorized into four groups based on body mass index (BMI); normal weight (BMI 18.5–24.9 kg/m^2), underweight (BMI < 18.5 kg/m^2), overweight (BMI 25.0–29.9 kg/m^2), and obesity (BMI ≥ 30.0 kg/m^2). SBP; systolic blood pressure, DBP; diastolic blood pressure, LDL-C; low-density lipoprotein cholesterol, HDL-C; high-density lipoprotein cholesterol.

3.2. Body Mass Index Category and Stroke

In men, during a mean follow-up of 1269 ± 928 days, 17,221 total strokes, 14,901 ischemic strokes, and 2,943 hemorrhagic strokes occurred. The incidence (95% confidence interval) of total stroke, ischemic stroke, and hemorrhagic stroke was 32.5 (32.0–32.9), 28.1 (27.6–28.5), and 5.5 (5.3–5.7) per 10,000 person-years in men. In women, during a mean follow-up of 1091 ± 893 days, 9159 total strokes, 8041 ischemic strokes, and 1443 hemorrhagic strokes occurred. The incidence (95% confidence interval) of total stroke, ischemic stroke, and hemorrhagic stroke was 25.7 (25.1–26.2), 22.5 (22.0–23.0), and 4.0 (3.8–4.2) per 10,000 person-years. Compared with the normal weight group, the incidence of total stroke and ischemic stroke was lower in the underweight group, whereas it was higher in the overweight and obese groups in both men and women. Compared with the normal weight group, the incidence of hemorrhagic stroke was lower in the underweight group, and higher in the overweight and obese groups in women. However, the incidence of the hemorrhagic group was higher in not only the overweight and obese groups, but also in the underweight group compared with the normal weight group in men. Multivariable Cox regression analyses showed that, compared with the normal weight group, overweight (HR 1.07, 95% CI 1.03–1.10) and obesity (HR 1.18, 95% CI 1.10–1.26) were associated with a higher incidence of total stroke in men. In women, compared with the normal weight group, overweight (HR 1.07, 95% CI 1.01–1.13) and obesity (HR 1.15, 95% CI 1.03–1.27) were also associated with a higher incidence of total stroke. In terms of ischemic stroke, overweight (HR 1.06, 95% CI 1.03–1.11) and obesity (HR 1.14, 95% CI 1.06–1.23) were associated with a higher risk than normal weight in men. Obesity was associated with a higher risk than normal weight in women (HR 1.13, 95% CI, 1.01–1.27). Notably, overweight, obesity, and underweight were not associated with the risk of hemorrhagic stroke in women. In men, overweight (HR 1.10, 95% CI 1.01–1.19) and obesity (HR 1.37, 95% CI 1.19–1.58) were associated with a greater risk of hemorrhagic stroke than normal weight. Furthermore, underweight was also associated with a higher risk (HR 1.58, 95% CI 1.30–1.91) (Table 2).

Table 2. Association between Body Mass Index Category and Stroke Events Stratified by Sex.

	Men				Women			
	Normal Weight (n = 1,013,302)	Underweight (n = 61,704)	Overweight (n = 382,425)	Obesity (n = 81,551)	Normal Weight (n = 832,491)	Underweight (n = 180,421)	Overweight (n = 146,243)	Obesity (n = 42,641)
	Total Stroke							
No. of events	10,608	455	5089	1069	6197	1108	1443	411
Incidence	29.9 (29.4–30.5)	24.2 (22.1–26.5)	38.7 (37.6–39.8)	41.5 (39.0–44.0)	24.8 (24.2–25.5)	20.3 (19.2–21.6)	34.7 (32.9–36.5)	35.8 (32.5–39.4)
Model 1	1 (Reference)	0.81 (0.74–0.89)	1.30 (1.25–1.34)	1.39 (1.31–1.48)	1 (Reference)	0.82 (0.77–0.87)	1.40 (1.32–1.48)	1.44 (1.31–1.59)
Model 2	1 (Reference)	0.97 (0.89–1.07)	1.25 (1.21–1.29)	1.67 (1.57–1.78)	1 (Reference)	0.97 (0.91–1.04)	1.20 (1.13–1.27)	1.45 (1.31–1.60)
Model 3	1 (Reference)	1.05 (0.95–1.15)	1.07 (1.03–1.10)	1.18 (1.10–1.26)	1 (Reference)	1.02 (0.95–1.08)	1.07 (1.01–1.13)	1.15 (1.03–1.27)
	Ischemic Stroke							
No. of events	9274	359	4395	873	5457	978	1257	349
Incidence	26.1 (25.6–26.7)	19.1 (17.2–21.1)	33.4 (32.4–34.4)	33.8 (31.6–36.1)	21.9 (21.3–22.4)	18.0 (16.9–19.1)	30.2 (28.6–31.9)	30.4 (27.4–33.7)
Model 1	1 (Reference)	0.73 (0.66–0.81)	1.28 (1.23–1.33)	1.30 (1.21–1.40)	1 (Reference)	0.82 (0.77–0.88)	1.38 (1.30–1.47)	1.39 (1.25–1.55)
Model 2	1 (Reference)	0.88 (0.79–0.98)	1.24 (1.19–1.28)	1.58 (1.47–1.69)	1 (Reference)	0.98 (0.91–1.05)	1.18 (1.11–1.26)	1.40 (1.25–1.55)
Model 3	1 (Reference)	0.95 (0.85–1.05)	1.06 (1.03–1.11)	1.14 (1.06–1.23)	1 (Reference)	1.02 (0.96–1.10)	1.06 (1.00–1.13)	1.13 (1.01–1.27)
	Hemorrhagic Stroke							
No. of events	1699	111	891	242	953	175	239	76
Incidence	4.8 (4.5–5.0)	5.9 (4.9–7.1)	6.7 (6.3–7.2)	9.3 (8.2–10.6)	3.8 (3.6–4.1)	3.2 (2.8–3.7)	5.7 (5.0–6.5)	6.6 (5.3–8.2)
Model 1	1 (Reference)	1.24 (1.02–1.50)	1.42 (1.30–1.53)	1.97 (1.72–2.26)	1 (Reference)	0.84 (0.72–0.99)	1.51 (1.31–1.74)	1.74 (1.38–2.20)
Model 2	1 (Reference)	1.45 (1.20–1.76)	1.36 (1.26–1.48)	2.21 (1.93–2.53)	1 (Reference)	0.96 (0.82–1.13)	1.33 (1.16–1.54)	1.72 (1.37–2.18)
Model 3	1 (Reference)	1.58 (1.30–1.91)	1.10 (1.01–1.19)	1.37 (1.19–1.58)	1 (Reference)	1.02 (0.87–1.20)	1.09 (0.94–1.26)	1.14 (0.89–1.45)

The incidence rate was per 10,000 person-years. Model 1 = Unadjusted, Model 2 = Adjusted for age, Model 3 = Adjusted for age, hypertension, diabetes mellitus, dyslipidemia, cigarette smoking, alcohol consumption, and physical inactivity.

3.3. Restricted Cubic Spline

Figure 2 shows the dose–response relationship between BMI and the risk of incident stroke. The association between BMI and the incidence of stroke was modeled using multivariable-adjusted spline regression models with a reference point set at BMI of 23 kg/m^2. A linear dose–response relationship was observed between BMI and the risk of total stroke in men (Figure 2A). In women, RCS showed that the risk of total stroke was lowest at around 20 kg/m^2 and increased in a dose-dependent manner after the BMI exceeded 20 kg/m^2 (Figure 2A). There was a linear dose–response relationship between BMI and the risk of ischemic stroke in men (Figure 2B). In women, RCS showed that the incidence of ischemic stroke was lowest at around 20 kg/m^2 and increased linearly after BMI exceeded approximately 20 kg/m^2 (Figure 2B). There was a U-shaped relationship between BMI and the risk of hemorrhagic stroke with the bottoms of splines around 23–24 kg/m^2 in men (Figure 2C). A dose-dependent association between BMI and the risk of hemorrhagic stroke was not evident in women (Figure 2C).

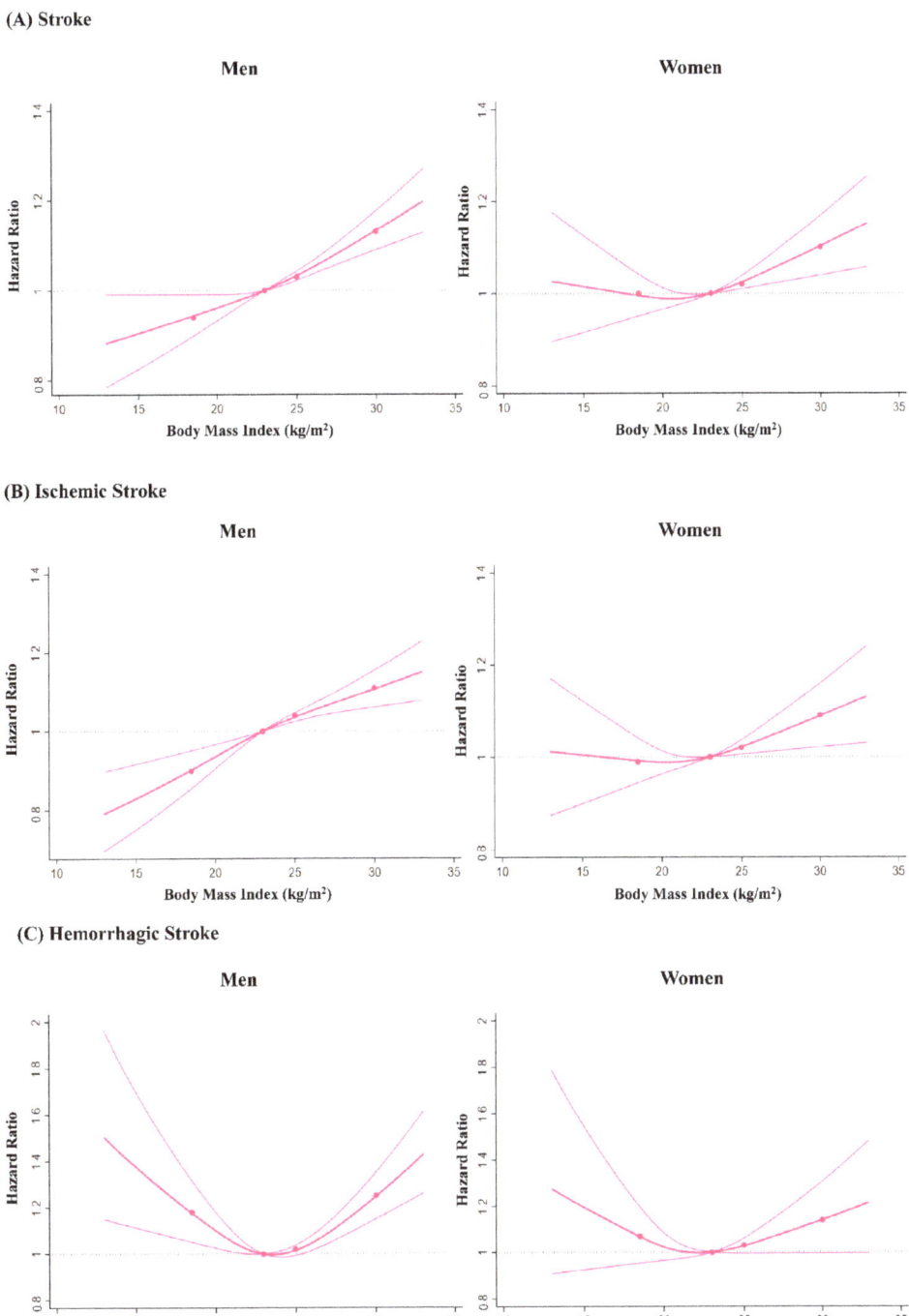

Figure 2. Restricted Cubic Spline. Restricted cubic spline of body mass index for total stroke (**A**), ischemic stroke (**B**), and hemorrhagic stroke (**C**).

3.4. Multiple Imputation for Missing Data

We analyzed 3,455,798 participants (1,996,118 men and 1,459,680 women) after multiple imputations for missing data. Among these participants, 22,444 and 11,273 total stroke events occurred in men and women, respectively. In this model, overweight and obesity were associated with a higher incidence of total stroke and ischemic stroke in both men and women. Both obesity and underweight were associated with a greater risk of hemorrhagic stroke in men, but not in women (Table 3).

Table 3. Association between Body Mass Index Category and Stroke Events Stratified by Sex after Multiple Imputation for Missing Data.

	Men				Women			
	Normal Weight (n = 1,321,093)	Underweight (n = 83,425)	Overweight (n = 487,325)	Obesity (n = 104,275)	Normal Weight (n = 1,012,062)	Underweight (n = 220,072)	Overweight (n = 175,854)	Obesity (n = 51,692)
	Total Stroke							
No. of events	13,772	612	6672	1388	7602	1375	1786	510
Incidence	28.4 (27.9–28.8)	22.4 (20.7–24.3)	37.9 (37.0–38.9)	40.0 (37.9–42.2)	24.5 (24.0–25.1)	20.2 (19.2–21.3)	34.8 (33.2–36.5)	35.6 (32.7–38.9)
Model 1	1 (Reference)	0.79 (0.73–0.86)	1.34 (1.30–1.38)	1.42 (1.34–1.50)	1 (Reference)	0.83 (0.78–0.87)	1.42 (1.35–1.50)	1.46 (1.33–1.59)
Model 2	1 (Reference)	0.99 (0.91–1.07)	1.26 (1.23–1.30)	1.66 (1.58–1.76)	1 (Reference)	0.98 (0.93–1.04)	1.21 (1.15–1.28)	1.44 (1.32–1.58)
Model 3	1 (Reference)	1.06 (0.98–1.15)	1.08 (1.05–1.11)	1.18 (1.12–1.25)	1 (Reference)	1.03 (0.97–1.09)	1.07 (1.02–1.13)	1.13 (1.03–1.24)
	Ischemic Stroke							
No. of events	12,015	494	5787	1131	6690	1209	1554	437
Incidence	24.7 (24.3–25.2)	18.1 (16.6–19.8)	32.9 (32.0–33.7)	32.5 (30.7–34.5)	21.6 (21.1–22.1)	17.8 (16.8–18.8)	30.3 (28.8–31.8)	30.5 (27.8–33.5)
Model 1	1 (Reference)	0.73 (0.67–0.80)	1.33 (1.29–1.37)	1.32 (1.24–1.41)	1 (Reference)	0.82 (0.78–0.88)	1.40 (1.33–1.48)	1.42 (1.29–1.56)
Model 2	1 (Reference)	0.92 (0.84–1.00)	1.25 (1.22–1.29)	1.57 (1.48–1.67)	1 (Reference)	0.98 (0.93–1.05)	1.20 (1.13–1.26)	1.41 (1.28–1.55)
Model 3	1 (Reference)	0.98 (0.90–1.07)	1.08 (1.05–1.12)	1.14 (1.07–1.21)	1 (Reference)	1.03 (0.97–1.10)	1.07 (1.01–1.13)	1.13 (1.02–1.25)
	Hemorrhagic Stroke							
No. of events	2253	139	1132	312	1189	220	301	91
Incidence	4.6 (4.4–4.8)	5.1 (4.3–6.0)	6.4 (6.0–6.8)	8.9 (8.0–10.0)	3.8 (3.6–4.0)	3.2 (2.8–3.7)	5.8 (5.2–6.5)	6.3 (5.1–7.8)
Model 1	1 (Reference)	1.10 (0.93–1.31)	1.39 (1.29–1.49)	1.95 (1.73–2.19)	1 (Reference)	0.84 (0.73–0.98)	1.53 (1.35–1.74)	1.66 (1.34–2.06)
Model 2	1 (Reference)	1.33 (1.12–1.58)	1.31 (1.22–1.41)	2.17 (1.92–2.44)	1 (Reference)	0.97 (0.84–1.12)	1.35 (1.19–1.53)	1.64 (1.32–2.02)
Model 3	1 (Reference)	1.44 (1.21–1.71)	1.06 (0.98–1.14)	1.37 (1.21–1.55)	1 (Reference)	1.02 (0.89–1.18)	1.09 (0.96–1.25)	1.06 (0.85–1.33)

The incidence rate was per 10,000 person-years. Model 1 = Unadjusted, Model 2 = Adjusted for age, Model 3 = Adjusted for age, hypertension, diabetes mellitus, dyslipidemia, cigarette smoking, alcohol consumption, and physical inactivity.

3.5. Non-Hypertensive Participants

After excluding hypertensive participants, we analyzed 1,199,658 men and 1,060,380 women in this model. Among them, 9310 and 6619 total stroke events occurred in men and women, respectively. Overweight and obesity were associated with a higher risk of total stroke or ischemic stroke in both men and women. Overweight and underweight were associated with a greater risk of hemorrhagic stroke in men. Notably, overweight, obesity, and underweight were not associated with a risk of hemorrhagic stroke in women (Table 4).

Table 4. Association between Body Mass Index Category and Stroke Events Stratified by Sex in Non-Hypertensive Participants.

	Men				Women			
	Normal Weight (n = 844,494)	Underweight (n = 57,301)	Overweight (n = 257,245)	Obesity (n = 40,618)	Normal Weight (n = 753,667)	Underweight (n = 172,343)	Overweight (n = 109,299)	Obesity (n = 25,071)
	Total Stroke							
No. of events	6508	320	2203	279	4730	943	793	153
Incidence	22.0 (21.5–22.6)	18.3 (16.4–20.5)	24.9 (23.8–25.9)	22.1 (19.7–24.9)	20.8 (20.2–21.4)	18.1 (16.9–19.2)	25.3 (23.6–27.1)	22.9 (19.5–26.8)
Model 1	1 (Reference)	0.84 (0.75–0.94)	1.13 (1.08–1.19)	1.02 (0.90–1.15)	1 (Reference)	0.87 (0.81–0.93)	1.22 (1.13–1.31)	1.10 (0.94–1.30)
Model 2	1 (Reference)	0.97 (0.87–1.09)	1.14 (1.09–1.20)	1.32 (1.17–1.49)	1 (Reference)	0.99 (0.92–1.06)	1.13 (1.05–1.22)	1.26 (1.07–1.48)
Model 3	1 (Reference)	0.99 (0.88–1.10)	1.09 (1.04–1.15)	1.20 (1.06–1.35)	1 (Reference)	1.00 (0.93–1.08)	1.09 (1.01–1.18)	1.20 (1.02–1.41)
	Ischemic Stroke							
No. of events	5785	253	1958	249	4222	840	709	142
Incidence	19.6 (19.1–20.1)	14.5 (12.8–16.4)	22.1 (21.1–23.1)	19.8 (17.5–22.4)	18.6 (18.0–19.2)	16.1 (15.0–17.2)	22.6 (21.0–24.4)	21.2 (18.0–25.0)
Model 1	1 (Reference)	0.75 (0.66–0.85)	1.13 (1.08–1.19)	1.02 (0.90–1.16)	1 (Reference)	0.87 (0.80–0.93)	1.22 (1.13–1.32)	1.15 (0.97–1.36)
Model 2	1 (Reference)	0.87 (0.76–0.98)	1.15 (1.09–1.21)	1.34 (1.18–1.52)	1 (Reference)	0.99 (0.92–1.07)	1.13 (1.04–1.22)	1.31 (1.11–1.55)
Model 3	1 (Reference)	0.88 (0.77–1.00)	1.09 (1.04–1.15)	1.21 (1.07–1.38)	1 (Reference)	1.01 (0.94–1.09)	1.09 (1.00–1.18)	1.24 (1.05–1.47)
	Hemorrhagic Stroke							
No. of events	902	78	316	37	643	135	110	12
Incidence	3.0 (2.8–3.2)	4.5 (3.6–5.6)	3.6 (3.2–4.0)	2.9 (2.1–4.0)	2.8 (2.6–3.0)	2.6 (2.2–3.1)	3.5 (2.9–4.2)	1.8 (1.0–3.1)
Model 1	1 (Reference)	1.48 (1.18–1.87)	1.17 (1.03–1.33)	0.98 (0.71–1.37)	1 (Reference)	0.91 (0.76–1.10)	1.25 (1.02–1.53)	0.64 (0.36–1.13)
Model 2	1 (Reference)	1.68 (1.34–2.12)	1.17 (1.03–1.33)	1.16 (0.84–1.61)	1 (Reference)	1.01 (0.84–1.21)	1.17 (0.96–1.43)	0.70 (0.39–1.23)
Model 3	1 (Reference)	1.66 (1.32–2.10)	1.15 (1.01–1.31)	1.12 (0.81–1.57)	1 (Reference)	0.99 (0.83–1.20)	1.18 (0.97–1.45)	0.71 (0.40–1.27)

The incidence rate was per 10,000 person-years. Model 1 = Unadjusted, Model 2 = Adjusted for age, Model 3 = Adjusted for age, diabetes mellitus, dyslipidemia, cigarette smoking, alcohol consumption, and physical inactivity.

4. Discussion

The current analyses using a nationwide epidemiological database including approximately 2,700,000 people without a prevalent history of CVD, demonstrated that overweight and obesity were associated with a greater risk of total stroke and ischemic stroke in both men and women. Furthermore, underweight was associated with a greater incidence of hemorrhagic stroke in men, but not in women. These results did not change after multiple imputations for missing data or excluding hypertensive participants.

Various studies have been conducted to explore the relationship between BMI and future stroke events [10–12]. Prospective studies including approximately 900,000 people showed that the mortality due to stroke increased in a dose-dependent manner with baseline BMI after it exceeded 25 kg/m^2 [28]. A population-based case–control study including 1,201 patients with ischemic stroke and 1154 controls aged 15–49 years showed that obesity defined as BMI > 30 kg/m^2 was associated with an increased risk (odds ratio, 1.57; 95% CI, 1.28–1.94) [29]. Additionally, a higher BMI in adolescents was associated with a greater risk of ischemic stroke [30]. The analysis of the Atherosclerosis Risk in Communities (ARIC) Study including approximately 13,000 black and white people showed that obesity was associated with a greater risk of ischemic stroke irrespective of race [31]. Ischemic stroke was a major subtype of total stroke [1,32], and the majority of the studies focused on the relationship between BMI and ischemic stroke. However, there have been several studies on the association between BMI and hemorrhagic stroke. A recent analysis of the China National Stroke Screening and Intervention Program showed that obesity was associated with a higher risk of total and ischemic stroke, whereas underweight was associated with an elevated risk of hemorrhagic stroke [16]. An analysis of 234,863 Korean men aged 40–64 years reported a positive association between BMI and incident ischemic stroke, whereas a J-shaped association was observed between BMI and hemorrhagic stroke [17].

Our results were generally in line with previous studies, as described above. The present study had several strengths. First, this study included a large number of participants without a prior history of CVD. Additionally, the JMDC Claims Database included the medical claims records from employees' insurance programs. Therefore, as long as each individual remained under coverage of the same insurance, the JMDC Claims Database could track the individuals' clinical information, including the diagnosis of stroke events, even if the individual visits different medical institutions. Second, sex differences are important in the risk stratification and prevention of CVD, including stroke. Furthermore, the value of BMI is different between sexes; therefore, we separately analyzed men and women. The positive association of overweight/obesity with the incidence of total stroke and ischemic stroke was consistent in both men and women. However, underweight was associated with a higher incidence of hemorrhagic stroke only in men. Therefore, there could be a gender difference in the relationship between BMI and incident stroke, particularly hemorrhagic stroke. Although similar findings were reported in a previous study including Korean men [17], data including men in the United States did not show an increase in the risk of hemorrhagic stroke in individuals having lower BMI [10]. A previous study including 39,053 women in the United States examined the relationship between BMI and incident stroke and showed that BMI was a risk factor for total or ischemic stroke but not for hemorrhagic stroke, and this relationship was attenuated after adjustment for hypertension, diabetes mellitus, and hypercholesterolemia [12]. Compared with this study including women in the United States, the relationship between BMI and incident stroke (particularly ischemic stroke) was seemingly more obvious even after adjustment for covariates in women of this study. Therefore, further investigations are required to verify our results. However, these associations in men and women did not change after multiple imputations for missing data. Furthermore, because hypertension is known to be a strong risk factor for both ischemic and hemorrhagic stroke, we conducted a sensitivity analysis after excluding hypertensive participants. Even in this model, the main results did not change. Third, because the association between BMI and incident stroke could change depending on the cut-off value of BMI for underweight, overweight, and obesity, we conducted the RCS of BMI for incident stroke to deal with BMI as a continuous value. Similar to the association of overweight, obesity, and underweight with the risk of stroke, RCS demonstrated a dose-dependent increase in the risk of total stroke and ischemic stroke with BMI in men and women, and a U-shaped relationship between BMI and future hemorrhagic stroke risk in men. These results suggest a potential difference in the association of BMI with risk of future events between ischemic and hemorrhagic stroke, particularly in men.

This study has several limitations. Due to the nature of retrospective observational studies, our study could not conclude a causal relationship between baseline BMI and incident stroke. For example, our study showed that overweight and obesity were associated with an elevated risk of ischemic stroke. However, whether body weight loss could reduce the future risk of ischemic stroke in overweight or obese participants could not be discussed in this study. Similarly, although underweight was associated with a greater incidence of hemorrhagic stroke in men, the underlying mechanism for this association and the optimal management strategy for this population should be elucidated in future studies. For example, malnutrition and specific comorbidities may contribute to the elevated incidence of hemorrhagic stroke in underweight participants. However, the JMDC Claims Database does not include sufficient data to consider this point. Although the incidence of CVD in this database is acceptable compared with other epidemiological data in Japan, the recorded diagnoses of administrative databases are generally considered less well-validated. Since the JMDC Claims Database primarily included an employed population of working age, a selection bias (e.g., healthy worker bias) might exist. Therefore, further investigations are needed to determine whether our findings can be expanded to other populations of different races, ethnicities, and socioeconomic status. The main results did not change after multiple imputations for missing data. However, the substantial proportion of missing data should be considered a major study limitation. Although we used BMI in this study, dual energy X-ray absorptiometry is a standard method to evaluate a body composition including fat. This discrepancy might have contributed to the wide confidence intervals at high and low BMI levels on the RCS curve in women. Data on medication status were limited in this study. For example, use of antithrombotic medication or statin could influence the results. However, we were unable to analyze these data. Although the change in mediation status could also influence the results, data on the change in medication status were not available in this study.

In conclusion, we analyzed a nationwide epidemiological database including a general population of 2,740,778 individuals with no prevalent history of CVD and found that overweight and obesity were associated with a higher incidence of total stroke and ischemic stroke in both sexes. Underweight was associated with a greater risk of future hemorrhagic stroke events in men, but not in women. Similarly, RCS showed that the risk of ischemic stroke dose-dependently increased with BMI in men and women, whereas there was a U-shaped relationship between BMI and future hemorrhagic stroke risk in men. Our results suggest that the association of BMI with subsequent risk differs between ischemic and hemorrhagic stroke, particularly in men.

Author Contributions: (1) Conception and design: H.K. (Hidehiro Kaneko), M.S., and I.K. (2) Analysis of data: M.S., H.I., K.M., S.M., H.K. (Hiroyuki Kiriyama), T.K., K.F., N.M., T.J., and H.Y. (3) Interpretation of data: H.K. (Hidehiro Kaneko), M.S., A.O., H.M., K.N., H.Y., and I.K. (4) Drafting of the manuscript: H.K. (Hidehiro Kaneko), M.S., and H.Y. (5) Critical revision for important intellectual content: N.T., H.M., S.N., and K.N. All authors have read and agreed to the published version of the manuscript.

Funding: This work was supported by grants from the Ministry of Health, Labour and Welfare, Japan (21AA2007) and the Ministry of Education, Culture, Sports, Science and Technology, Japan (20H03907, 21H03159, and 21K08123). The funding sources had nothing with regard to the current study.

Institutional Review Board Statement: This study was conducted according to the ethical guidelines of our institution (approval by the Ethical Committee of The University of Tokyo: 2018–10862) and in accordance with the principles of the Declaration of Helsinki. The requirement for in-formed consent was waived because all the data from the JMDC Claims Database were de-identified.

Informed Consent Statement: The requirement for in-formed consent was waived because all the data from the JMDC Claims Database were de-identified.

Data Availability Statement: The data from the JMDC Claims Database are available for anyone who would purchase it from JMDC Inc. (JMDC Inc.; Tokyo, Japan; https://www.jmdc.co.jp/en/index), which is a healthcare venture company in Tokyo, Japan.

Conflicts of Interest: The authors declare no conflict of interest.

Disclosures

Research funding and scholarship funds (Hidehiro Kaneko and Katsuhito Fujiu) from Medtronic Japan CO., LTD, Boston Scientific Japan CO., LTD, Biotronik Japan, Simplex QUANTUM CO., LTD, and Fukuda Denshi, Central Tokyo CO., LTD.

Non-Standard Abbreviations and Acronyms

BMI	Body Mass Index
CI	Confidence Interval
CVD	Cardiovascular Disease
HR	Hazard Ratio
RCS	Restricted Cubic Spline

References

1. Virani, S.S.; Alonso, A.; Benjamin, E.J.; Bittencourt, M.S.; Callaway, C.W.; Carson, A.P.; Chamberlain, A.M.; Chang, A.R.; Cheng, S.; Delling, F.N.; et al. Heart Disease and Stroke Statistics-2020 Update: A Report from the American Heart Association. *Circulation* **2020**, *141*, e139–e596. [CrossRef]
2. Feigin, V.L.; Nguyen, G.; Cercy, K.; Johnson, C.O.; Alam, T.; Parmar, P.G.; Abajobir, A.A.; Abate, K.H.; Abd-Allah, F.; Abejie, A.N.; et al. Global, Regional, and Country-Specific Lifetime Risks of Stroke, 1990 and 2016. *N. Engl. J. Med.* **2018**, *379*, 2429–2437.
3. Feigin, V.L.; Mensah, G.A.; Norrving, B.; Murray, C.J.; Roth, G.A.; GBD 2013 Stroke Panel Experts Group. Atlas of the Global Burden of Stroke (1990–2013): The GBD 2013 Study. *Neuroepidemiology* **2015**, *45*, 230–236. [CrossRef] [PubMed]
4. Timmis, A.; Townsend, N.; Gale, C.P.; Torbica, A.; Lettino, M.; Petersen, S.E.; Mossialos, E.A.; Maggioni, A.P.; Kazakiewicz, D.; May, H.T.; et al. European Society of Cardiology: Cardiovascular Disease Statistics 2019. *Eur. Heart J.* **2020**, *41*, 12–85. [CrossRef]
5. Guh, D.P.; Zhang, W.; Bansback, N.; Amarsi, Z.; Birmingham, C.L.; Anis, A.H. The incidence of co-morbidities related to obesity and overweight: A systematic review and meta-analysis. *BMC Public Health* **2009**, *9*, 88. [CrossRef]
6. Hubert, H.B.; Feinleib, M.; McNamara, P.M.; Castelli, W.P. Obesity as an independent risk factor for cardiovascular disease: A 26-year follow-up of participants in the Framingham Heart Study. *Circulation* **1983**, *67*, 968–977. [CrossRef]
7. Poirier, P.; Giles, T.D.; Bray, G.A.; Hong, Y.; Stern, J.S.; Pi-Sunyer, F.X.; Eckel, R.H. Obesity and cardiovascular disease: Pathophysiology, evaluation, and effect of weight loss: An update of the 1997 American Heart Association Scientific Statement on Obesity and Heart Disease from the Obesity Committee of the Council on Nutrition, Physical Activity, and Metabolism. *Circulation* **2006**, *113*, 898–918.
8. Yusuf, S.; Hawken, S.; Ounpuu, S.; Bautista, L.; Franzosi, M.G.; Commerford, P.; Lang, C.C.; Rumboldt, Z.; Onen, C.L.; Lisheng, L.; et al. Obesity and the risk of myocardial infarction in 27,000 participants from 52 countries: A case-control study. *Lancet* **2005**, *366*, 1640–1649. [CrossRef]
9. Calle, E.E.; Thun, M.J.; Petrelli, J.M.; Rodriguez, C.; Heath, C.W., Jr. Body-mass index and mortality in a prospective cohort of U.S. adults. *N. Engl. J. Med.* **1999**, *341*, 1097–1105. [CrossRef] [PubMed]
10. Kurth, T.; Gaziano, J.M.; Berger, K.; Kase, C.S.; Rexrode, K.M.; Cook, N.R.; Buring, J.E.; Manson, J.E. Body mass index and the risk of stroke in men. *Arch Intern Med.* **2002**, *162*, 2557–2562. [CrossRef]
11. Yatsuya, H.; Toyoshima, H.; Yamagishi, K.; Tamakoshi, K.; Taguri, M.; Harada, A.; Ohashi, Y.; Kita, Y.; Naito, Y.; Yamada, M.; et al. Body mass index and risk of stroke and myocardial infarction in a relatively lean population: Meta-analysis of 16 Japanese cohorts using individual data. *Circ. Cardiovasc. Qual. Outcomes* **2010**, *3*, 498–505. [CrossRef]
12. Kurth, T.; Gaziano, J.M.; Rexrode, K.M.; Kase, C.S.; Cook, N.R.; Manson, J.E.; Buring, J.E. Prospective study of body mass index and risk of stroke in apparently healthy women. *Circulation* **2005**, *111*, 1992–1998. [CrossRef]
13. Senoo, K.; Nakata, M.; Teramukai, S.; Kumagai, M.; Yamamoto, T.; Nishimura, H.; Lip, G.Y.H.; Matoba, S. Relationship Between Body Mass Index and Incidence of Atrial Fibrillation in Young Japanese Men- The Nishimura Health Survey. *Circ. J.* **2021**, *85*, 243–251. [CrossRef] [PubMed]
14. Itoh, H.; Kaneko, H.; Kiriyama, H.; Kamon, T.; Fujiu, K.; Morita, K.; Yotsumoto, H.; Michihata, N.; Jo, T.; Takeda, N.; et al. Reverse J-shaped relationship between body mass index and in-hospital mortality of patients hospitalized for heart failure in Japan. *Heart Vessel.* **2021**, *36*, 383–392. [CrossRef] [PubMed]
15. Echouffo-Tcheugui, J.B.; Masoudi, F.A.; Bao, H.; Curtis, J.P.; Heidenreich, P.A.; Fonarow, G.C. Body mass index and outcomes of cardiac resynchronization with implantable cardioverter-defibrillator therapy in older patients with heart failure. *Eur. J. Heart Fail.* **2019**, *21*, 1093–1102. [CrossRef]
16. Qi, W.; Ma, J.; Guan, T.; Zhao, D.; Abu-Hanna, A.; Schut, M.; Chao, B.; Wang, L.; Liu, Y. Risk Factors for Incident Stroke and Its Subtypes in China: A Prospective Study. *J. Am. Heart Assoc.* **2020**, *9*, e016352. [CrossRef]
17. Song, Y.M.; Sung, J.; Davey Smith, G.; Ebrahim, S. Body mass index and ischemic and hemorrhagic stroke: A prospective study in Korean men. *Stroke* **2004**, *35*, 831–836. [CrossRef] [PubMed]
18. Kaneko, H.; Itoh, H.; Yotsumoto, H.; Kiriyama, H.; Kamon, T.; Fujiu, K.; Morita, K.; Michihata, N.; Jo, T.; Morita, H.; et al. Association of body weight gain with subsequent cardiovascular event in non-obese general population without overt cardiovascular disease. *Atherosclerosis* **2020**, *308*, 39–44. [CrossRef]
19. Goto, A.; Goto, M.; Terauchi, Y.; Yamaguchi, N.; Noda, M. Association Between Severe Hypoglycemia and Cardiovascular Disease Risk in Japanese Patients with Type 2 Diabetes. *J. Am. Heart Assoc.* **2016**, *5*, e002875. [CrossRef]
20. Wake, M.; Onishi, Y.; Guelfucci, F.; Oh, A.; Hiroi, S.; Shimasaki, Y.; Teramoto, T. Treatment patterns in hyperlipidaemia patients based on administrative claim databases in Japan. *Atherosclerosis* **2018**, *272*, 145–152. [CrossRef]
21. Kawasaki, R.; Konta, T.; Nishida, K. Lipid-lowering medication is associated with decreased risk of diabetic retinopathy and the need for treatment in patients with type 2 diabetes: A real-world observational analysis of a health claims database. *Diabetes Obes. Metab.* **2018**, *20*, 2351–2360. [CrossRef]
22. Kaneko, H.; Itoh, H.; Kiriyama, H.; Kamon, T.; Fujiu, K.; Morita, K.; Michihata, N.; Jo, T.; Takeda, N.; Morita, H.; et al. Lipid Profile and Subsequent Cardiovascular Disease among Young Adults Aged <50 Years. *Am. J. Cardiol.* **2021**, *142*, 59–65.
23. Kaneko, H.; Itoh, H.; Yotsumoto, H.; Kiriyama, H.; Kamon, T.; Fujiu, K.; Morita, K.; Kashiwabara, K.; Michihata, N.; Jo, T.; et al. Cardiovascular Health Metrics of 87,160 Couples: Analysis of a Nationwide Epidemiological Database. *J. Atheroscler. Thromb.* **2020**, *28*, 535–543. [CrossRef] [PubMed]

24. Kaneko, H.; Itoh, H.; Kamon, T.; Fujiu, K.; Morita, K.; Michihata, N.; Jo, T.; Morita, H.; Yasunaga, H.; Komuro, I. Association of Cardiovascular Health Metrics with Subsequent Cardiovascular Disease in Young Adults. *J. Am. Coll. Cardiol.* **2020**, *76*, 2414–2416. [CrossRef] [PubMed]
25. Yagi, M.; Yasunaga, H.; Matsui, H.; Morita, K.; Fushimi, K.; Fujimoto, M.; Koyama, T.; Fujitani, J. Impact of Rehabilitation on Outcomes in Patients with Ischemic Stroke: A Nationwide Retrospective Cohort Study in Japan. *Stroke* **2017**, *48*, 740–746. [CrossRef] [PubMed]
26. Aloisio, K.M.; Swanson, S.A.; Micali, N.; Field, A.; Horton, N.J. Analysis of partially observed clustered data using generalized estimating equations and multiple imputation. *Stata J.* **2014**, *14*, 863–883. [CrossRef]
27. Rubin, D.B.; Schenker, N. Multiple imputation in health-care databases: An overview and some applications. *Stat. Med.* **1991**, *10*, 585–598. [CrossRef]
28. Prospective Studies Collaboration; Whitlock, G.; Lewington, S.; Sherliker, P.; Clarke, R.; Emberson, J.; Halsey, J.; Qizilbash, N.; Collins, R.; Peto, R. Body-mass index and cause-specific mortality in 900,000 adults: Collaborative analyses of 57 prospective studies. *Lancet* **2009**, *373*, 1083–1096. [PubMed]
29. Mitchell, A.B.; Cole, J.W.; McArdle, P.F.; Cheng, Y.C.; Ryan, K.A.; Sparks, M.J.; Mitchell, B.D.; Kittner, S.J. Obesity increases risk of ischemic stroke in young adults. *Stroke* **2015**, *46*, 1690–1692. [CrossRef]
30. Bardugo, A.; Fishman, B.; Libruder, C.; Tanne, D.; Ram, A.; Hershkovitz, Y.; Zucker, I.; Furer, A.; Gilon, R.; Chodick, G.; et al. Body Mass Index in 1.9 Million Adolescents and Stroke in Young Adulthood. *Stroke* **2021**, *52*, 2043–2052. [CrossRef]
31. Yatsuya, H.; Folsom, A.R.; Yamagishi, K.; North, K.E.; Brancati, F.L.; Stevens, J.; Atherosclerosis Risk in Communities Study Investigators. Race- and sex-specific associations of obesity measures with ischemic stroke incidence in the Atherosclerosis Risk in Communities (ARIC) study. *Stroke* **2010**, *41*, 417–425. [CrossRef] [PubMed]
32. Krishnamurthi, R.V.; Feigin, V.L.; Forouzanfar, M.H.; Mensah, G.A.; Connor, M.; Bennett, D.A.; Moran, A.E.; Sacco, R.L.; Anderson, L.M.; Truelsen, T.; et al. Global and regional burden of first-ever ischaemic and haemorrhagic stroke during 1990–2010: Findings from the Global Burden of Disease Study 2010. *Lancet Glob. Health* **2013**, *1*, e259–e281. [CrossRef]

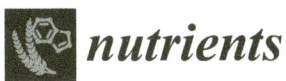

Article

Omega-3 Fatty Acids in Erythrocyte Membranes as Predictors of Lower Cardiovascular Risk in Adults without Previous Cardiovascular Events

Gustavo Henrique Ferreira Gonçalinho, Geni Rodrigues Sampaio, Rosana Aparecida Manólio Soares-Freitas and Nágila Raquel Teixeira Damasceno *

Department of Nutrition, School of Public Health, University of São Paulo, São Paulo 01246-904, Brazil; ghfg93@gmail.com (G.H.F.G.); genirs@usp.br (G.R.S.); rosanaso@usp.br (R.A.M.S.-F.)
* Correspondence: nagila@usp.br; Tel.: +55-11-3061-7865; Fax: +55-11-3061-7721

Abstract: *Background*: This study investigated the association of omega-3 polyunsaturated fatty acids (*n*-3 PUFA) within erythrocyte membranes and cardiovascular risk assessed by three different estimates. *Methods*: Inclusion criteria were individuals of both sexes, 30 to 74 years, with at least one cardiovascular risk factor, and no previous cardiovascular events (*n* = 356). Exclusion criteria were individuals with acute or chronic severe diseases, infectious diseases, pregnant, and/or lactating women. Plasma biomarkers (lipids, glucose, and C-reactive protein) were analyzed, and nineteen erythrocyte membrane fatty acids (FA) were identified. The cardiovascular risk was estimated by Framingham (FRS), Reynolds (RRS), and ACC/AHA-2013 Risk Scores. Three patterns of FA were identified (Factor 1, poor in *n*-3 PUFA), (Factor 2, poor in PUFA), and (Factor 3, rich in *n*-3 PUFA). *Results*: Total cholesterol was inversely correlated with erythrocyte membranes C18:3 *n*-3 (r = −0.155; *p* = 0.004), C22:6 *n*-3 (r = −0.112; *p* = 0.041), and total *n*-3 (r = −0.211; *p* < 0.001). Total *n*-3 PUFA was associated with lower cardiovascular risk by FRS (OR = 0.811; 95% CI= 0.675–0.976). Regarding RRS, Factor 3 was associated with 25.3% lower odds to have moderate and high cardiovascular risk (OR = 0.747; 95% CI = 0.589–0.948). The ACC/AHA-2013 risk score was not associated with isolated and pooled FA. *Conclusions*: *n*-3 PUFA in erythrocyte membranes are independent predictors of low-risk classification estimated by FRS and RRS, which could be explained by cholesterol-lowering effects of *n*-3 PUFA.

Keywords: *n*-3 polyunsaturated fatty acids; cardiovascular risk estimates; cardiovascular diseases; biomarkers; cardiovascular risk factors

Citation: Gonçalinho, G.H.F.; Sampaio, G.R.; Soares-Freitas, R.A.M.; Damasceno, N.R.T. Omega-3 Fatty Acids in Erythrocyte Membranes as Predictors of Lower Cardiovascular Risk in Adults without Previous Cardiovascular Events. *Nutrients* 2021, *13*, 1919. https://doi.org/10.3390/nu13061919

Academic Editors: Carlo Agostoni and Hayato Tada

Received: 22 April 2021
Accepted: 26 May 2021
Published: 3 June 2021

Publisher's Note: MDPI stays neutral with regard to jurisdictional claims in published maps and institutional affiliations.

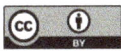

Copyright: © 2021 by the authors. Licensee MDPI, Basel, Switzerland. This article is an open access article distributed under the terms and conditions of the Creative Commons Attribution (CC BY) license (https://creativecommons.org/licenses/by/4.0/).

1. Introduction

Cardiovascular diseases (CVD) remain the major cause of death worldwide. Therefore, the assessment and monitoring of cardiovascular (CV) risk through algorithms has shown to be an accurate tool to predict outcomes, as well as to improve treatment indication when compared with the isolated use of risk factors [1–3]. The estimates use risk factors that are the major contributors to cardiovascular events (i.e., age, sex, glycemia, blood pressure, and blood lipids) [3–5]. The ten-years CV risk estimation is relevant especially in moderate-risk patients because the intuitive ten-year period is important in making practical and usually therapeutic, decisions. Cardiovascular risk assessment models have been built to guide the treatment of modified cardiovascular risk factors and, in the last decade to help therapeutic goals based on statins. Moreover, the estimates provide insight into the individual contribution of variables to the patient's risk, guiding the preventive care [1]. However, the application of these estimates requires previous validation for the target population. Many CV risk estimates were developed based on American or European white populations, and the estimation of multi-ethnic populations is often overestimated [6–9].

Nevertheless, the Framingham Risk Score (FRS) is the most popular estimating tool and its use is currently recommended by many guidelines, including in Brazil [10].

Omega-3 polyunsaturated fatty acids (n-3 PUFA) are often highlighted due to several mechanisms that modify CV risk factors, slow down the atherosclerotic process and, possibly change cardiovascular events. The eicosapentaenoic (EPA; C20:5 n-3) and docosahexaenoic acids (DHA; C22:6 n-3) are the main components of this family, is often linked to antiarrhythmic effects, autonomic function improvement, decreased platelet aggregation, vasodilatory effects, blood pressure reduction, endothelial function improvement, atherosclerotic plaque stabilization, increased adiponectin synthesis, reduction of collagen deposition in the arteries, anti-inflammatory effects, and reduction of plasma triglycerides and cholesterol, consequently reducing CVD risk [11]. Despite that, reports of randomized trials have shown small or even null effects on cardiovascular risk factors and outcomes [12].

Most of the studies show methodological differences and do not assess n-3 PUFA biomarkers. Circulating or tissue n-3 PUFA have proven their superiority in estimating habitual intake compared to dietary assessment [13]. Based on that, previous studies have associated n-3 PUFA in erythrocyte membranes with reduced CV risk and mortality [13–16]. Because n-3 PUFA alter some components included in CV risk estimates, it is possible to state that n-3 PUFA influence the overall CV risk which is frequently used to guide preventive care. Thus, the nutritional status of n-3 PUFA may be useful in CVD prevention. However, as far as it is known, no previous study investigated the association of isolated and clustered FA biomarkers with different cardiovascular risk estimates.

Therefore, the main goal of this study was to investigate the association of erythrocyte membranes n-3 PUFA with different cardiovascular risk estimate classifications in Brazilian individuals. In addition, we also evaluated the association of modified CV risk factors used in estimates with isolated and clusters n-3 PUFA.

2. Materials and Methods

2.1. Study Design and Participants

This was a cross-sectional study, using the baseline data from the CARDIONUTRI clinical trial (ReBEC: RBR-2vfhfv), which included individuals from the outpatient clinic at the University Hospital of the University of São Paulo. The study selection was made public by poster, newspaper, and digital media (sites, electronic mailing, and social networks). Inclusion criteria were individuals of both sexes, 30 to 74 years, with at least one cardiovascular risk factor, and no previous cardiovascular events. Exclusion criteria were individuals with acute or chronic severe diseases, infectious diseases, pregnant, and/or lactating women. Individuals interested in participating in the study were submitted to a short phone interview to assess inclusion and exclusion criteria. Additionally, individuals were submitted to electrocardiogram assessment by a trained physician, and those with alterations suggesting previous cardiovascular events were excluded. Three hundred and seventy-four individuals were recruited for the study from 2011–2012. Two individuals declined after clarification of the study design. Fourteen were excluded due to altered electrocardiogram and one due to recent HIV diagnosis. At the end of the recruitment, 356 individuals were included in the study.

2.2. Clinical, Physical Activity, and Diet Assessment

Sociodemographic status, lifestyle, family history of chronic diseases, self-report of non-communicable chronic diseases, and current medication use were investigated through questionnaires. Physical examination included body mass index (BMI) assessment and blood pressure levels. Dietary intake was obtained through three 24 h-recalls and assessed in the Food Processor software (ESHA Research, 2012), with subsequent energy adjustment [17]. A physical activity questionnaire validated for the Brazilian population was applied [18–20]. This questionnaire investigates the habitual physical activity (divided into physical exercise in leisure, leisure, and locomotion activities and total physical activity score) performed in the last 12 months, associated with frequency, duration, intensity. Baecke's physical activity scores do not allow to classify physical activity, however, for each one of its sixteen questions, the points vary from 0 (zero) to 5. The final score is directly proportional to physical activity and is useful to associate with health outcomes [18–20].

2.3. Biochemical Measurements

Blood was drawn after a 12-h fast, placed in EDTA tubes (1.0 mg/mL), and erythrocytes were separated from plasma by centrifugation, and both were frozen at −80 °C immediately after collection. Protease inhibitors (10 µg/mL of aprotinin, 10 µg/mL of benzamidine and 5 µg/mL of phenylmethylsulfonyl fluoride) and BHT (100 µg/mL) were added to preserve samples. All samples were divided into aliquots to avoid repeated defrost cycles and storage at −80 °C until analyses. Plasma total cholesterol, HDL-c, TG, glucose (Labtest Diagnostica SA, MG, Brazil), Apo A-I and Apo B (Wako Chemicals USA Inc., Richmond, VA, USA), and high sensitivity C-reactive protein (hs-CRP) (Diagnostic System Laboratories, Inc., Webster, TX, USA) were measured by commercial kits. LDL-c was calculated according to the Friedewald equation.

2.4. Erythrocyte Fatty Acids Analysis

The analysis of FA from erythrocyte membranes was performed based on a previous method [21]. After plasma separation (3000× g, 10 min, 4 °C), 300 µL of erythrocytes were washed with 5 mL of phosphate-buffered saline (PBS) solution (pH 7.4) four times. The precipitate was transferred to threaded tubes, to which 1.75 mL of methanol, 50 µL of an internal standard solution containing 1 mg tridecanoic acid (C13:0)/1 mL hexane, and 100 µL of acetyl chloride were added. Thereafter, the solution was vortexed and heated in a water bath at 90 °C for 1 h. After that, 1.5 mL of hexane was added, and the solution was homogenized for 1 min. The samples were centrifuged at 1500× g, 4 °C for 2 min, and 800 µL of the supernatant was transferred to a different tube. This step was repeated with the addition of 750 µL of hexane. The tubes containing the collected supernatants were placed on a centrifugal concentrator at 40 °C for 20 min. Then the FA methyl esters were dissolved in 150 µL of hexane and transferred to a glass insert in a vial. Analyses were conducted considering the fatty acids individually, as well as the total n-3 (C18:3 n-3 + C20:3 n-3 + 20:5 n-3 + C22:5 n-3 + 22:6 n-3), total n-6 (C18:2 n-6 + C20:4 n-6) and Omega-3 Index (C20:5 n-3 + C22:6 n-3), the latter having been named by Harris and von Schacky [13]. To assess biological effects of fatty acids, the following ratios were calculated: C20:4 n-6/C20:5 n-3, C18:3 n-3/C20:5 n-3, C18:3 n-3/C22:6 n-3 and C18:2 n-6/C18:3 n-3.

2.5. Cardiovascular Risk Assessment

The CV risk was assessed by FRS [1,22], Reynolds Risk Score (RRS) [23,24], and the American College of Cardiology/American Heart Association 2013 Risk Score (ACC/AHA-2013) [25]. The CV risk was stratified into three categories for each score: low, moderate, and high risk. Diabetes (i.e., glucose ≥ 126 mg/dL or current hypoglycemic medication use) was considered a coronary artery disease (CAD) equivalent [26].

2.6. Statistical Analysis

Distribution of variables was assessed through the Kolmogorov-Smirnov test. Sample characteristics are presented as mean and standard deviation (SD) or median and interquartile range (IQR) depending on the variable's distribution. For categorical variables, results are shown in absolute value (n) and its percentage (%). Spearman's and Pearson's correlations were applied to evaluate associations between cardiovascular risk factors and FA.

Kappa (k) agreement analysis was performed between ACC/AHA 2013, FRS, and RRS to verify the agreement between the cardiovascular risk stratifications, and the strength of agreement was classified according to Landis and Koch (1977) [27].

A factor analysis was performed to establish the patterns of erythrocyte membranes FA composition to subsequently associate them with CV risk. It is a multivariate statistical analysis for the identification of factors in a set of measurements [28]. Sample adequacy was checked using the Kaiser-Meyer-Olklin (KMO) index and Barlett's test of sphericity. KMO values > 0.50 and $p < 0.05$ were considered acceptable. The choice of the number of factors was based on eigenvalues > 1.0 and scree plot analysis. Factor loadings were analyzed after orthogonal rotation using the varimax method. The considered threshold of factor loadings was 0.2. Negative loadings indicated that FA were inversely associated with the corresponding factor, just as positive loadings indicated a direct association [28]. Three factors were generated.

To further evaluate potential confounders of the associations between erythrocyte membranes FA and CV risk estimates, multiple linear and logistic regressions were applied using baseline sample characteristics as covariates (age, sex, race, schooling, smoking, systolic blood pressure, BMI, glucose, triglycerides, total cholesterol, HDL-c, C-reactive protein, physical activity, drinking habits, treatments with statins, antihypertensives, fibrates, and hypoglycemic drugs, family history of myocardial infarction, obesity, hypertension, and stroke) and total n-3 and n-6 PUFA, Factor 1, Factor 2 and Factor 3 as dependent variables. Assumptions for linear regression such as lack of multicollinearity of predictors, residuals' homoscedasticity and normality, linearity, and independence were evaluated. n-6 PUFA, Factor 1, and Factor 3 covered all assumptions, while total n-3 and Factor 2 presented nonparametric residuals. Thus, linear regressions were not applied to these latter variables. The multiple linear regressions were applied using the backwards method, and final models were presented. Multiple logistic regressions were applied to total n-3 PUFA and Factor 2 (categorized by median) using the backwards-likelihood ratio method and models with the best correct classification were chosen.

Logistic regressions were used with CV risk scores as dependent variables (0 = low CV risk and 1 = moderate and high CV risk) and FA or Factors as independent variables. Because age, race, sex, total cholesterol, HDL-c, SBP, glucose, and C-reactive protein are covariates already entered into the equations of the CV risk estimates, these were not used as adjustments of the regressions. All regressions were adjusted by physical activity, BMI, and education level. Since there is no data on socioeconomic status, a known predictor of CV risk, education level was used as an adjustment in the models [29].

The missing data was handled by pairwise methods [30]. All tests were two-sided, considered significant when $p < 0.05$, and performed using the software Stata version 14 and SPSS version 20.

3. Results

The characteristics of the individuals (n = 356) are summarized in Table 1. The mean age was 52.5 (10.4) years old (men = 49.4 years and women = 54.4 years; $p < 0.001$) and 62.6% were women. It was observed a high frequency of hypertension (57%) and a family history of the disease (65.2%). In addition, 51.7% of the individuals were on antihypertensive treatment. Most individuals were classified as a high cardiovascular risk by FRS (52.2%) and ACC/AHA 2013 score (50.4%), while only 29.1% classified by RRS show similar risk levels. The mean BMI was 30.9 (5.8) Kg/m^2. Current smoking (26.3% vs. 15.7%; $p = 0.003$) and alcohol intake (64.7% vs. 35%; $p < 0.001$) were more frequent in men. As expected, for all cardiovascular risk estimates men and women showed significant differences (Table S1). Table 2 describes the biochemical and clinical profile of individuals. The mean total cholesterol level was 205.0 (42.6) mg/dL. The mean CRP was 2.8 (1.2–6.0 mg/L). Dyslipidemia (53.9%) and hypertension (57.0%) were highly prevalent. When individuals were compared by sex, women showed higher total cholesterol, LDL-c, and CRP than men, while HDL-c and Apo A-I were higher (Table S2).

Although women had a higher intake of total lipids, eicosatrienoic (C20:3 n-3) and docosapentaenoic (C22:5 n-3) than men, the 19 FA in erythrocyte membranes presented in Table 3 did not show differences between sexes (Table S3). Fourteen from nineteen FA identified met the criteria for factorial analysis model (KMO = 0.632; Barlett's Test of

Sphericity < 0.001). Factor 1 was rich in *n*-6 PUFA and poor in *n*-3 PUFA, Factor 2 was poor in PUFA, and Factor 3 was rich in *n*-3 PUFA and poor in *n*-6 PUFA (Table S4).

Table 1. Demographic and clinical characterization of individuals.

Variables	n	Total
Age (years)	356	52.5 (10.4)
Ethnicity (n, %)	356	
White		238 (66.9)
Non-white		118 (33.1)
Smoking (n, %)	356	
Current smoker		70 (19.7)
Non-smoker		286 (80.3)
Alcohol consumption (n, %)	356	
Yes		164 (46.1)
No		192 (53.9)
Education (n, %)		
High school or less		208 (58.4)
College		148 (41.6)
Chronic non-communicable diseases (n, %)	356	
Diabetes Mellitus		72 (20.2)
Hypertension		203 (57.0)
Hypothyroidism		43 (12.1)
Dyslipidemia		192 (53.9)
Medication (n, %)	356	
Statins		98 (27.5)
Antihypertensives		184 (51.7)
Hypoglycemic		74 (20.8)
Fibrates		9 (2.5)
Family history of diseases (n, %)	356	
Obesity		64 (18.0)
Hypertension		232 (65.2)
Myocardial infarction		100 (28.1)
Stroke		68 (19.1)
Diabetes Mellitus		134 (37.6)
Physical activity (points)		7.18 (1.39)
Framingham Risk Score (n,%)	356	
Low risk		43 (12.1)
Moderate risk		127 (35.7)
High risk		186 (52.2)
Reynolds Risk Score (n,%)	351	
Low risk		154 (43.9)
Moderate risk		95 (27.1)
High risk		102 (29.1)
ACC/AHA-2013 Risk Score (n,%)	355	
Low risk		130 (36.6)
Moderate risk		46 (13.0)
High risk		179 (50.4)

Continuous variables are shown as mean (standard deviation) or median (interquartile range), and categorical data as n (%). BMI: body mass index; SBP: systolic blood pressure; DBP: diastolic blood pressure; TG: triglycerides; LDL-c: low density lipoprotein-cholesterol, HDL-c: high density lipoprotein-cholesterol.

Total cholesterol was inversely correlated with erythrocyte membranes C18:3 *n*-3 ($r = -0.155$; $p = 0.004$), C22:6 *n*-3 ($r = -0.112$; $p = 0.041$), Omega-3 Index ($r = -0.124$; $p = 0.023$) and total *n*-3 ($r = -0.211$; $p < 0.001$), and positively correlated with total *n*-6 ($r = 0.178$; $p = 0.001$) and Factor 1 ($r = 0.170$; $p = 0.002$), which is rich in *n*-6 PUFA and poor in *n*-3 PUFA (Table S5). Multivariate linear and logistic regressions were applied to evaluate the associations between the covariates entered in CV risk estimates, baseline characteristics and erythrocyte membranes *n*-3 and *n*-6 PUFA to verify potential confounding factors (Tables S6 and S7). Total cholesterol, BMI, triglycerides, family history of obesity, and age were independently associated with erythrocyte membranes FA (Tables S6 and S7).

Figure 1 shows the CV risk classification and its concordance. The most frequent stratification of CV risk assessment by RRS was low CV risk (n = 154; 43.9%), whilst ACC/AHA 2013 and FRS were the scores that classified most individuals as high risk (n = 179; 50.4% and n = 186; 52.2%, respectively). The agreement of cardiovascular risk stratifications obtained through estimates was modest. The agreement between FRS and RRS was 51% (k = 0.30, p < 0.001), and there was a moderate agreement between FRS and ACC/AHA 2013, of 64% (k = 0.43, p < 0.001) and between ACC/AHA 2013 and RRS, with 67% (k = 0.50, p < 0.001). Based on that, all CV risk estimates were maintained in the next analyses.

Table 2. Biochemical and clinical characterization of individuals.

Variables	n	Total
SBP (mmHg)	356	133 (18.0)
DBP (mmHg)		81 (10.0)
Hypertension ($\geq$140 mmHg) (n, %)	356	111 (31.2)
BMI (kg/m^2)	356	30.9 (5.8)
Obesity (BMI $\geq$ 30.0 kg/m^2) (n, %)		182 (51.1)
Total cholesterol (mg/dL)	354	205.0 (42.6)
Hypercholesterolemia ($\geq$200mg/dL) (n, %)		193 (54.2)
LDL-c (mg/dL)	340	137.3 (38.7)
High LDL-c ($\geq$130 mg/dL) (n, %)		196 (55.1)
HDL-c (mg/dL)	354	36.0 (30.0–42.3)
Low-HDL-c (<40 mg/dL) (n, %)		125 (35.1)
Triglycerides (mg/dL)	354	130.5 (98.0–191.3)
Hypertriglyceridemia ($\geq$150 mg/dL) (n, %)		145 (40.7)
Glucose (mg/dL)	354	98.0 (91.0–108.0)
Hyperglycemia ($\geq$100 mg/dL) (n, %)		164 (46.1)
Apo A-I (mg/dL)	355	132.2 (25.7)
Low-Apo A-I (<120 mg/dL) (n, %)		230 (64.6)
Apo B (mg/dL)	355	104.7 (24.8)
High-Apo B ($\geq$120 mg/dL) (n, %)		88 (24.7)
C-reactive protein (mg/L)	347	2.84 (1.2–6.0)
High-CRP (>1.0 mg/L) (n, %)		275 (77.2)

Categorical variables are shown as absolute value (n) and frequency (%). Continuous variables are shown as mean (standard deviation) or median (interquartile range). BMI: body mass index; SBP: systolic blood pressure; DBP: diastolic blood pressure; TG: triglycerides; LDL-c: low density lipoprotein-cholesterol, HDL-c: high density lipoprotein-cholesterol.

The Table 4 describes the association of CV scores estimates and erythrocytes membranes FA. The regression analyses showed that each unit increase of C18:3 n-3 was associated with 20.8% odds reduction of being classified as intermediate or high risk (OR = 0.792; 95% CI = 0.635–0.988). Each unit increase of total n-3 PUFA (C18:3 n-3 + C20:5 n-3 + C22:6 n-3) had 20.2% odds increase of low CV risk classification by FRS (OR = 0.798; 95% CI = 0.672–0.946). There were also 2.8% odds increase of low CV risk classification regarding the C18:3 n-3/C20:5 n-3 ratio (OR = 0.972; 95% CI = 0.945–1.000). Each unit increase of n-6/n-3 and C18:2 n-6/C18:3 n-3 ratios were associated with 47.3% (OR = 1.473; 95% CI = 1.021–2.126) and 27.6% (OR = 1.276; 95% CI = 1.043–1.561) odds increase of intermediate or high CV risk classification, respectively. After adjustment, only total n-3 PUFA remained statistically significant (OR = 0.811; 95% CI = 0.675–0.976).

Factor 1 (rich in n-6 PUFA) was associated with odds increase of intermediate or high CV risk classification by 40.8% by FRS (OR = 1.408; 95% CI = 1.036–1.913). After adjustment, the odds increased to 46.9% (OR = 1.469; 95% CI = 1.056–2.043) by FRS and 27.6% by RRS (OR = 1.276; 95% CI: 1.010–1.612). Factor 3 (rich in n-3 PUFA) was associated with odds increase of low CV risk classification by 26.6% according to RRS (OR = 0.734; 95% CI = 0.585–0.921). After adjustment, the odds increased by 25.3% (OR = 0.747; 95% CI = 0.589–0.948). Erythrocyte membranes FA and membranes patterns were not statistically significant associated with the ACC/AHA 2013 risk score (Table S8).

Table 3. Erythrocyte membranes fatty acids profile (n = 335).

Variables	Total
SFA (%)	
C16:0	43.6 (41.1–47.5)
C18:0	24.8 (22.9–27.3)
C20:0	0.7 (0.6–0.8)
C22:0	1.1 (0.9–1.4)
C24:0	0.3 (0.1–0.7)
MUFA (%)	
C16:1 n-7	0.3 (0.2–0.6)
C18:1 n-9	10.0 (3.5)
C20:1 n-9	0.0 (0.1–0.1)
C22:1 n-9	0.1 (0.1–0.2)
C24:1 n-9	1.3 (0.5)
PUFA n-6 (%)	
C18:2 n-6	4.7 (1.8)
C18:3 n-6	0.2 (0.1–0.2)
C20:2 n-6	0.1 (0.1–0.2)
C20:3 n-6	0.6 (0.3)
C20:4 n-6	2.5 (1.4–5.1)
C22:2 n-6	0.4 (0.3–0.6)
Total n-6	9.4 (3.8)
PUFA n-3 (%)	
C18:3 n-3	0.2 (0.1–0.2)
C20:5 n-3	0.2 (0.1–0.3)
C22:6 n-3	3.4 (2.7–4.2)
Omega-3 Index	3.6 (3.0–4.5)
Total n-3	5.7 (4.8–6.7)
Fatty acids ratios	
C16:0/C16:1 n-7	130.7 (67.9–232.6)
C18:0/C18:1 n-9	2.5 (2.0–3.4)
n-6/n-3	1.7 (1.0–2.4)
C20:4 n-6/C20:5 n-3	12.9 (5.6–27.6)
C18:3 n-3/C20:5 n-3	9,1 (5.7–14.0)
C18:2 n-6/C20:4 n-6	1.8 (1.0–2.8)
C18:2 n-6/C18:3 n-3	2.4 (1.4–4.2)

SFA: saturated fatty acids; PUFA: polyunsaturated fatty acids; MUFA: monounsaturated fatty acids. Omega-3 Index: C20:5 n-3 + C22:6 n-3. Total n-3: C18:3 n-3 + 20:5 n-3+ 22:6. n-6: C18:2 n-6 + C18:3 n-6 + C20:2 n-6 + C20:3 n-6 + C20:4 n-6 + C22:2 n-6. Data are shown as mean (standard deviation) or median (interquartile range) depending on the distribution.

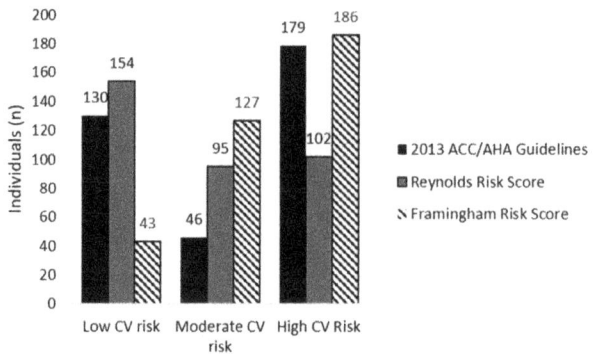

	ACC/AHA 2013	FRS	RRS
ACC/AHA 2013	-	64% (0.43)*	67% (0.50)*
FRS	64% (0.43)*	-	51% (0.30)*
RRS	67% (0.50)*	51% (0.30)*	-

Figure 1. Distribution and agreement of global cardiovascular risk stratifications between different predictive equations. Data are shown in % agreement and kappa values. *: p-value < 0.001.

Table 4. Logistic regression models of isolated and pooled erythrocyte membranes fatty acids and FRS and RRS.

Fatty Acids	Framingham Risk Score				Reynolds Risk Score			
	Unadjusted Model		Adjusted Model *		Unadjusted Model		Adjusted Model *	
	OR	CI (95%)	OR	CI (95%)	OR	CI (95%)	OR	CI (95%)
C18:3 n-3	0.792	**0.635–0.988**	0.819	0.642–1.046	0.911	0.766–1.082	0.925	0.772–1.108
C20:5 n-3	5.016	0.409–61.557	6.176	0.374–102.027	0.417	0.095–1.835	0.378	0.078–1.823
C22:6 n-3	0.830	0.655–1.052	0.833	0.654–1.062	1.033	0.867–1.232	1.033	0.861–1.239
Total n-3	0.798	**0.672–0.946**	0.811	**0.675–0.976**	0.959	0.842–1.091	0.968	0.845–1.108
Total n-6	1.077	0.986–1.176	1.079	0.984–1.183	1.033	0.975–1.094	1.049	0.987–1.115
Omega-3 index	0.840	0.660–1.069	0.844	0.660–1.079	1.021	0.855–1.220	1.020	0.849–1.226
n-6/n-3	1.473	**1.021–2.126**	1.421	0.972–2.078	1.099	0.886–1.363	1.117	0.890–1.403
C20:4 n-6/C20:5 n-3	1.002	0.986–1.020	1.002	0.985–1.020	1.005	0.994–1.016	1.008	0.996–1.019
C18:3 n-3/C20:5 n-3	0.972	**0.945–1.000**	0.973	0.945–1.003	0.989	0.966–1.012	0.990	0.966–1.014
C18:3 n-3/C22:6 n-3	0.764	0.455–1.285	0.856	0.482–1.521	0.888	0.599–1.317	0.923	0.613–1.391
C18:2 n-6/C18:3 n-3	1.276	**1.043–1.561**	1.229	0.995–1.518	0.995	0.980–1.009	0.988	0.970–1.006
Factor 1	1.408	**1.036–1.913**	1.469	**1.056–2.043**	1.208	0.969–1.507	1.276	**1.010–1.612**
Factor 2	1.577	0.878–2.831	1.516	0.812–2.832	1.099	0.876–1.378	1.087	0.860–1.375
Factor 3	0.923	0.671–1.271	0.992	0.697–1.411	0.734	**0.585–0.921**	0.747	**0.589–0.948**

*: model adjusted by body mass index (BMI), physical activity and education level. Omega-3 Index: C20:5 n-3 + C22:6 n-3. Total n-3: C18:3 n-3 + 20:5 n-3 + 22:6 n-3; total n-6: C18:2 n-6 + C18:3 n-6 + C20:2 n-6 + C20:3 n-6 + C20:4 n-6 + C22:2 n-6. Odds ratio (OR) per unit change of FA. The bold highlights statistically significant associations.

4. Discussion

The findings of the study show that a higher content of *n*-3 PUFA in erythrocyte membranes was associated with higher odds of CV risk being classified as low. Unlike prior studies, the patterns of erythrocyte membranes FA composition were investigated, and the results corroborate the cardioprotective associations of *n*-3 PUFA.

CV risk estimates do not allow to establish a causal relationship with cardiovascular events and mortality but are useful for healthcare professionals to monitor interventions focused on modifying classic risk factors and to further assess individual patient risk. Regarding the effects of *n*-3 PUFA on CV risk factors by multiple direct and indirect mechanisms, it is plausible to assume it influences the estimated CV risk as proposed by previous studies. In 50 cases with acute non-fatal MI and 50 age- and sex-matched controls without MI the Omega-3 Index was significantly lower in cases than in controls (9.57% (SEM = 0.28) vs. 11.81% (SEM = 0.35); $p < 0.001$) in addition to the decreased risk of non-fatal MI (OR = 0.08; 95% CI = 0.02–0.38). Also, a CV risk estimate based on the FA profile (sum of C20:5 *n*-3, C18:3 *n*-3, *trans*-oleic acid, and C20:4 *n*-6) showed a higher contribution to the discrimination of MI cases compared to controls when compared to FRS, being a potential predictor of outcomes [31]. The similar way, a study evaluating MI 2-year mortality showed that the red blood cells (RBC) FA C20:5 *n*-3 and C22:5 *n*-6 of 1144 patients changed the *c*-statistic of the GRACE score from 0.747 ($p < 0.001$) to 0.768 ($p < 0.05$ vs. GRACE alone), improved the net reclassification index by 31% (95% CI = 15–48%) and the relative incremental discrimination index by 19.8% (95% CI = 7.5–35.7%). Those results show that RBC FA improved the prediction of 2-year mortality over the GRACE score in MI patients [32]. In the present study, two patterns of erythrocyte membranes FA composition were associated with CV risk classification. The pattern rich in *n*-3 PUFA (Factor 3) increased the odds of low-risk classification by 25.3% by RRS, whilst the pattern rich in *n*-6 PUFA (Factor 1) increased the odds of moderate or high-risk classification by 46.9% and 27.6% by FRS and RRS, respectively.

Studies have shown inverse associations between *n*-3 PUFA biomarkers and CVD. Two meta-analyses have shown associations of *n*-3 PUFA biomarkers from different compartments with coronary risk reduction [14,15]. In a cohort, C20:5 *n*-3, C22:6 *n*-3, and Omega-3 Index in erythrocyte membranes were inversely associated with CV mortality, with stronger results when C20:5 *n*-3 was higher than 1% [33]. In several populations, the Omega-3 Index is associated with reduced coronary risk [13,34,35]. Recently, in the Framingham Offspring Cohort, individuals with Omega-3 Index higher than 6.8% had 39% fewer cardiovascular events compared to those in which the index was lower than 4.2%. Another finding of this study was 59% and 32% lower risks of stroke and all-cause mortality in individuals with C22:6 *n*-3 higher than 5.96% when compared to those lower than 3.69% [16]. The present study did not identify a significant association of the Omega-3 Index and CV risk classifications; however, robust associations were observed for C18:3 *n*-3 and total *n*-3 with lower CV risk estimated by FRS and pooled FA rich in *n*-3 (Factor 3) and RRS. Conversely, Factor 1 (rich in *n*-6), and total *n*-6/*n*-3 and C18:2 *n*-6/C18:3 *n*-3 ratios modified the previous association, reducing the benefits attributed to FA *n*-3. This profile can be explained by the reduced content of the Omega-3 Index (<4%) in 62.7% of the participants, whereas 36.4% had a sub-optimal content (4% to 8%), with only 0.9% showing an optimal level, according to Omega-3 Index classification proposed by Harris & von Schacky [13].

The complex relationship of FA and CV risk estimates may be partially explained by associations between C18:3 *n*-3, C22:6 *n*-3, and total *n*-3 PUFA and total cholesterol, suggesting that the associations with CV risk classification are related to the cholesterol-lowering effect of *n*-3 PUFA. Zibaeenezhad et al. evaluated the impact of fresh fish intake (250 g/week) and fish oil supplementation (2 g/day) during 8 weeks on lipid profile. The consumption of dietary fish has shown better effect on the reduction of total cholesterol and LDL-c compared with fish oil [36]. Although the positive effect of *n*-3 on hypertriglyceridemia (from 25% to 30% triglycerides reduction) is a consensus in literature [37], the isolated effect on total cholesterol and LDL-c remains controversial. Two systematic reviews based on fish intake, EPA-containing capsules, and algae DHA oil confirm the positive effect of n-3 PUFA on the reduction of triglycerides without changes in LDL-c [38,39]. Contrary, Wei et al. (2011) observed a 5% LDL-c increase after DHA intake, while EPA decreased by 1% [40]. Together, these results indicate that n-3 PUFA modulates lipid profile by multiple mechanisms, which contributes to association with better CV risk classification observed in the present study.

The three CV risk estimates tested in this study were validated in American Caucasians, and the application on different populations without validation may overestimate the risk. Although the Brazilian population is multi-ethnic, the Brazilian Society of Cardiology guidelines recommends using FRS for CV risk estimation [10]. The ACC/AHA 2013 risk score is currently recommended by America Heart Association guidelines [25], and the RRS had a better prediction compared to FRS in the American population, in addition to considering family history and inflammation in the equation [23,24]. The ACC/AHA 2013 risk score has shown good calibration and discrimination in an American cohort [9], but its application in and European population indicated 96.4% of men and 65.8% of women classified as high risk [6]. In the multi-centric cohort Multi-Ethnic Study of Atherosclerosis (MESA), containing 6814 individuals self-referred as Caucasians, Blacks, Hispanics, or Chinese, the ACC/AHA 2013 risk score had the worst calibration and discrimination compared to FRS, RRS, and ATP-III Risk Score, overestimating risk for both men (154%) and women (67%), with an overall disagreement of 115% [7]. In turn, FRS overestimated men's risk in 37% and women's risk in 8%, with an overall disagreement of 25%, whilst RRS overestimated men's risk in only 9%, and underestimated women's risk in 21%, in addition to showing the slightest overall disagreement (−3%) [7]. In Women's Health Initiative Observational Cohort, FRS overestimated the risk and had worse calibration and discrimination compared to RRS [8]. In the MESA cohort, RRS also outperformed FRS in predicting subclinical atherosclerosis assessed by coronary artery calcification (CAC), an important predictor of CV risk, through computerized tomography [41]. Those studies suggest that ACC/AHA 2013 risk score and FRS overestimate risk in multi-ethnic populations, and the frequency of high-risk stratifications in this study corroborates with them. The agreement analyses performed in this study confirm the differences between these CV risk estimates. Although FRS and ACC/AHA 2013 consider the same parameters to estimate the CV risk, the subtle differences in both algorithms may explain the modest agreement between them and subsequently, the absence of association of n-3 PUFA and ACC/AHA 2013 observed in this study.

Furthermore, it important to highlight that despite the highest agreement between ACC/AHA 2013 and RRS (67%; k = 0.50), due to the high frequency of low-risk classifications, the first estimate does not consider the inflammation in CV risk. We hypothesized that because the CRP is a component of RRS and is modulated by n-3 PUFA, it would strengthen the association between both variables. However, no associations between CRP and n-3 PUFA were found in the study. Previous studies show a strong relationship between n-3 PUFA and CRP. In 2019, the study of Omar et al. showed that high intake of n-3 (2.0 g/day) reduced blood lipids (total cholesterol, LDL-c, and triglycerides) and inflammatory markers such as interleukin-6 and CRP [42]. Similar results were observed when purified eicosapentaenoic acid ethyl ester (4.0 g/day) was used in ANCHOR study, in which a significant reduction in triglycerides and CRP, without changing LDL-c [43].

Certainly, the most relevant limitation of our results is the lack of information about CV outcomes. Another limitation was the lack of socioeconomic status data in the study, which is an important predictor of CV risk. Despite of that, education level, which was used as the adjustment, may reflect socioeconomic status as predictor of health [29]. Furthermore, the modifiable and non-modifiable risk factors considered in the CV risk estimates are not able to explain all cardiovascular events, so the CV outcome prediction may not reflect the real risk. Therefore, the effects of n-3 PUFA on CV risk may be underestimated due to mechanisms that act independently of traditional risk factors, such as platelet inhibition and arrhythmia reduction [11,44]. It is important to note that an important portion of the individuals in the study use medications that can affect the associations and mask the effects of PUFA on CV health, such as lipid-lowering drugs. For future studies regarding CV risk scores, a prescreening of individuals based on n-3 PUFA level could show more clearly the effects of n-3 PUFA on CV risk classification, although higher levels (>4%) of n-3 PUFA may not be frequent in Western countries due to low intake [35].

The strengths of this investigation include the application of FA biomarkers, being more objective than the traditional dietetic assessment. This study investigated not only single FA associations but the FA patterns through factor analysis. These patterns might depict the manifold biological interactions with FA, which the isolated analysis would not do. As far as it is known, this study is the first to assess erythrocyte membranes FA patterns through factor analysis. Moreover, the application of multiple CV risk estimates uses major CV risk factors and indirectly reflects the clinical outcomes, being useful in short-term or cross-sectional investigations.

5. Conclusions

In conclusion, the results of this study have shown that n-3 PUFA in erythrocyte membranes are associated with better CV risk classification estimated by FRS and RRS in Brazilian individuals, which could be explained by the cholesterol-lowering effects of n-3 PUFA.

Supplementary Materials: The following are available online at https://www.mdpi.com/article/10.3390/nu13061919/s1, Table S1: Demographic and clinical characterization of individuals, according to sex. Table S2: Biochemical profile of individuals, according to sex. Table S3: Erythrocyte membranes fatty acids, according to sex. Table S4: Factor loadings of fatty acids in erythrocyte membranes. Table S5: Correlations between erythrocyte membranes PUFA and variables used in cardiovascular risk estimates. Table S6: Multiple linear regressions associating baseline characteristics and erythrocyte membrane fatty acids. Table S7: Multiple logistic regressions associating baseline characteristics and erythrocyte membrane fatty acids. Table S8: Logistic regression models of isolated and pooled erythrocyte membranes fatty acids and ACC/AHA 2013 risk score.

Author Contributions: G.H.F.G. contributed to the biochemical and statistical analysis, critical review and writing; G.R.S. and R.A.M.S.-F. were responsible for biochemical analyses and draw of the tables and figure, and N.R.T.D. contributed to the study design, critical review and writing. All authors have read and agreed to the published version of the manuscript.

Funding: Grants received from Coordenação de Aperfeiçoamento de Pessoal de Nível Superior (CAPES n°88882.330835/2019-01), and grants received from State of Sao Paulo Research Foundation (FAPESP 2016/24531-3, 2011/12523-2).

Institutional Review Board Statement: This study was conducted according to the guidelines of the Declaration of Helsinki, and approved by the local Research Ethics Committee as register under number 0063.0.207.198-11.

Informed Consent Statement: All procedures were obtained only after all subjects to sign the informed consent.

Data Availability Statement: Full data can be asked to the corresponding author.

Acknowledgments: The authors cordially thank Elizabeth Torres for making the GC equipment available for analysis, João Valentini Neto and Adélia Pereira Neta for their support in the statistical analysis.

Conflicts of Interest: The authors declare no conflict of interest.

Ethics Committee: All procedures followed the rules established by the University of São Paulo University Hospital Research Ethics Committee as register under number 0063.0.207.198-11. All procedures were in accordance with the ethical standards of the institutional and/or national research committee and with the 1964 Helsinki declaration and its later amendments or comparable ethical standards.

References

1. D'Agostino, R.B.; Vasan, R.S.; Pencina, M.J.; Wolf, P.A.; Cobain, M.; Massaro, J.M.; Kannel, W.B. General cardiovascular risk profile for use in primary care: The Framingham heart study. *Circulation* **2008**, *117*, 743–753. [CrossRef]
2. DeGoma, E.M.; Dunbar, R.L.; Jacoby, D.; French, B. Differences in absolute risk of cardiovascular events using risk-refinement tests: A systematic analysis of four cardiovascular risk equations. *Atherosclerosis* **2013**, *227*, 172–177. [CrossRef] [PubMed]
3. Hardoon, S.L.; Whincup, P.H.; Lennon, L.T.; Wannamethee, S.G.; Capewell, S.; Morris, R.W. How much of the recent decline in the incidence of myocardial infarction in British men can be explained by changes in cardiovascular risk factors? Evidence from a prospective population-based study. *Circulation* **2008**, *117*, 598–604. [CrossRef]
4. Stamler, J.; Wentworth, D.; Neaton, J.D. Is Relationship Between Serum Cholesterol and Risk of Premature Death From Coronary Heart Disease Continuous and Graded?: Findings in 356 222 Primary Screenees of the Multiple Risk Factor Intervention Trial (MRFIT). *JAMA* **1986**, *256*, 2823–2828. [CrossRef] [PubMed]
5. Unal, B.; Critchley, J.A.; Capewell, S. Explaining the decline in coronary heart disease mortality in England and Wales between 1981 and 2000. *Circulation* **2004**, *109*, 1101–1107. [CrossRef]
6. Kavousi, M.; Leening, M.J.G.; Nanchen, D.; Greenland, P.; Graham, I.M.; Steyerberg, E.W.; Ikram, M.A.; Stricker, B.H.; Hofman, A.; Franco, O.H. Comparison of application of the ACC/AHA guidelines, Adult Treatment Panel III guidelines, and European Society of Cardiology guidelines for cardiovascular disease prevention in a European cohort. *JAMA* **2014**, *311*, 1416–1423. [CrossRef]
7. DeFilippis, A.P.; Young, R.; Carrubba, C.J.; McEvoy, J.W.; Budoff, M.J.; Blumenthal, R.S.; Kronmal, R.A.; McClelland, R.L.; Nasir, K.; Blaha, M.J. An analysis of calibration and discrimination among multiple cardiovascular risk scores in a modern multiethnic cohort. *Ann. Intern. Med.* **2015**, *162*, 266–275. [CrossRef]
8. Cook, N.R.; Paynter, N.P.; Eaton, C.B.; Manson, J.E.; Martin, L.W.; Robinson, J.G.; Rossouw, J.E.; Wassertheil-Smoller, S.; Ridker, P.M. Comparison of the framingham and reynolds risk scores for global cardiovascular risk prediction in the multiethnic women's health initiative. *Circulation* **2012**, *125*, 1748–1756. [CrossRef] [PubMed]
9. Muntner, P.; Colantonio, L.D.; Cushman, M.; Goff, D.C.; Howard, G.; Howard, V.J.; Kissela, B.; Levitan, E.B.; Lloyd-Jones, D.M.; Safford, M.M. Validation of the atherosclerotic cardiovascular disease Pooled Cohort risk equations. *JAMA* **2014**, *311*, 1406–1415. [CrossRef] [PubMed]
10. Faludi, A.A.; Izar, M.C.; Saraiva, J.F.; Chacra, A.P.; Bianco, H.T.; Afiune Neto, A.; Bertolami, A.; Pereira, A.C.; Lottenberg, A.M.; Sposito, A.C.; et al. Atualização da diretriz brasileira de dislipidemias e prevenção da aterosclerose—2017. *Arq. Bras. Cardiol.* **2017**, *109*, 76. [CrossRef]
11. Manson, J.E.; Cook, N.R.; Lee, I.-M.; Christen, W.; Bassuk, S.S.; Mora, S.; Gibson, H.; Albert, C.M.; Gordon, D.; Copeland, T.; et al. Marine n−3 Fatty Acids and Prevention of Cardiovascular Disease and Cancer. *N. Engl. J. Med.* **2019**, *380*, 23–32. [CrossRef] [PubMed]
12. Aung, T.; Halsey, J.; Kromhout, D.; Gerstein, H.C.; Marchioli, R.; Tavazzi, L.; Geleijnse, J.M.; Rauch, B.; Ness, A.; Galan, P.; et al. Associations of omega-3 fatty acid supplement use with cardiovascular disease risks meta-analysis of 10 trials involving 77 917 individuals. *JAMA Cardiol.* **2018**, *3*, 225–234. [CrossRef]
13. Harris, W.S.; Von Schacky, C. The Omega-3 Index: A new risk factor for death from coronary heart disease? *Prev. Med.* **2004**, *39*, 212–220. [CrossRef]
14. Chowdhury, R.; Warnakula, S.; Kunutsor, S.; Crowe, F.; Ward, H.A.; Johnson, L.; Franco, O.H.; Butterworth, A.; Forouhi, N.G.; Thompson, S.G.; et al. Association of dietary, circulating, and supplement fatty acids with coronary risk. *Ann. Intern. Med.* **2014**, *160*, 398–406. [CrossRef]
15. Del Gobbo, L.C.; Imamura, F.; Aslibekyan, S.; Marklund, M.; Virtanen, J.K.; Wennberg, M.; Yakoob, M.Y.; Chiuve, S.E.; Dela Cruz, L.; Frazier-Wood, A.C.; et al. ω-3 Polyunsaturated fatty acid biomarkers and coronary heart disease: Pooling project of 19 cohort studies. *JAMA Intern. Med.* **2016**, *176*, 1155–1166. [CrossRef]
16. Harris, W.S.; Tintle, N.L.; Etherton, M.R.; Vasan, R.S. Erythrocyte long-chain omega-3 fatty acid levels are inversely associated with mortality and with incident cardiovascular disease: The Framingham Heart Study. *J. Clin. Lipidol.* **2018**, *12*, 718–727. [CrossRef] [PubMed]
17. Willett, W.C.; Howe, G.R.; Kushi, L.H. Adjustment for total energy intake in epidemiologic studies. *Am. J. Clin. Nutr.* **1997**, *65*, 1220S–1228S. [CrossRef]
18. Baecke, J.A.; Burema, J.; Frijters, J.E. A short questionnaire for the measurement habitual physical activity in epidemiological studies. *Am. J. Clin. Nutr.* **1982**, *36*, 936–942. [CrossRef] [PubMed]
19. Florindo, A.A.; Latorre, M.; do, R.D.; de, O. Validation and reliability of the Baecke questionnaire for the evaluation of habitual physical activity in adult men. *Rev. Bras. Med. Esporte* **2003**, *9*, 129–135. [CrossRef]
20. Garcia, L.; Osti, R.; Ribeiro, E.; Florindo, A. Validação de dois questionários para a avaliação da atividade física em adultos. *Rev. Bras. Ativ. Física Saúde* **2013**, *18*. [CrossRef]
21. Masood, A.; Stark, K.D.; Salem, N. A simplified and efficient method for the analysis of fatty acid methyl esters suitable for large clinical studies. *J. Lipid Res.* **2005**, *46*, 2299. [CrossRef]
22. Mosca, L.; Benjamin, E.J.; Berra, K.; Bezanson, J.L.; Dolor, R.J.; Lloyd-Jones, D.M.; Newby, L.K.; Piña, I.L.; Roger, V.L.; Shaw, L.J.; et al. Effectiveness-based guidelines for the prevention of cardiovascular disease in women—2011 Update: A guideline from the American Heart Association. *J. Am. Coll. Cardiol.* **2011**, *57*, 1404–1423. [CrossRef]

23. Ridker, P.M.; Buring, J.E.; Rifai, N.; Cook, N.R. Development and validation of improved algorithms for the assessment of global cardiovascular risk in women: The Reynolds Risk Score. *J. Am. Med. Assoc.* **2007**, *297*, 611–619. [CrossRef]
24. Ridker, P.M.; Paynter, N.P.; Rifai, N.; Gaziano, J.M.; Cook, N.R. C-reactive protein and parental history improve global cardiovascular risk prediction: The Reynolds risk score for men. *Circulation* **2008**, *118*, 2243–2251. [CrossRef] [PubMed]
25. Goff, D.C.; Lloyd-Jones, D.M.; Bennett, G.; Coady, S.; D'Agostino, R.B.; Gibbons, R.; Greenland, P.; Lackland, D.T.; Levy, D.; O'Donnell, C.J.; et al. 2013 ACC/AHA guideline on the assessment of cardiovascular risk: A report of the American college of cardiology/American heart association task force on practice guidelines. *J. Am. Coll. Cardiol.* **2014**, *63*, 2935–2959. [CrossRef] [PubMed]
26. Catapano, A.L.; Reiner, Ž.; De Backer, G.; Graham, I.; Taskinen, M.R.; Wiklund, O.; Agewall, S.; Alegria, E.; Chapman, M.J.; Durrington, P.; et al. ESC/EAS Guidelines for the management of dyslipidaemias. The Task Force for the management of dyslipidaemias of the European Society of Cardiology (ESC) and the European Atherosclerosis Society (EAS). *Atherosclerosis* **2011**, *217*, 3–46. [CrossRef] [PubMed]
27. Landis, J.R.; Koch, G.G. The Measurement of Observer Agreement for Categorical Data. *Biometrics* **1977**, *33*, 159. [CrossRef] [PubMed]
28. Marchioni, D.M.L.; Latorre, M.; do, R.D.; de, O.; Eluf-Neto, J.; Wünsch-Filho, V.; Fisberg, R.M. Identification of dietary patterns using factor analysis in and epidemiological study in São Paulo. *São Paulo Med. J.* **2005**, *123*, 124–127. [CrossRef]
29. Winkleby, M.A.; Jatulis, D.E.; Frank, E.; Fortmann, S.P. Socioeconomic status and health: How education, income, and occupation contribute to risk factors for cardiovascular disease. *Am. J. Public Health* **1992**, *82*, 816–820. [CrossRef]
30. Kang, H. The prevention and handling of the missing data. *Korean J. Anesthesiol.* **2013**, *64*, 402–406. [CrossRef]
31. Park, Y.; Lim, J.; Lee, J.; Kim, S.G. Erythrocyte fatty acid profiles can predict acute non-fatal myocardial infarction. *Br. J. Nutr.* **2009**, *102*, 1355–1361. [CrossRef]
32. Harris, W.S.; Kennedy, K.F.; O'Keefe, J.H.; Spertus, J.A. Red blood cell fatty acid levels improve GRACE score prediction of 2-yr mortality in patients with myocardial infarction. *Int. J. Cardiol.* **2013**, *168*, 53–59. [CrossRef] [PubMed]
33. Kleber, M.E.; Delgado, G.E.; Lorkowski, S.; März, W.; von Schacky, C. Omega-3 fatty acids and mortality in patients referred for coronary angiography. The Ludwigshafen Risk and Cardiovascular Health Study. *Atherosclerosis* **2016**, *252*, 175–181. [CrossRef]
34. Block, R.C.; Harris, W.S.; Reid, K.J.; Sands, S.A.; Spertus, J.A. EPA and DHA in blood cell membranes from acute coronary syndrome patients and controls. *Atherosclerosis* **2008**, *197*, 821–828. [CrossRef]
35. Harris, W.S.; Del Gobbo, L.; Tintle, N.L. The Omega-3 Index and relative risk for coronary heart disease mortality: Estimation from 10 cohort studies. *Atherosclerosis* **2017**, *262*, 51–54. [CrossRef] [PubMed]
36. Zibaeenezhad, M.J.; Ghavipisheh, M.; Attar, A.; Aslani, A. Comparison of the effect of omega-3 supplements and fresh fish on lipid profile: A randomized, open-labeled trial. *Nutr. Diabetes* **2017**, *7*, 1. [CrossRef] [PubMed]
37. Din, J.N.; Harding, S.A.; Valerio, C.J.; Sarma, J.; Lyall, K.; Riemersma, R.A.; Newby, D.E.; Flapan, A.D. Dietary intervention with oil rich fish reduces platelet-monocyte aggregation in man. *Atherosclerosis* **2008**, *197*, 290–296. [CrossRef] [PubMed]
38. Balk, E.M.; Lichtenstein, A.H.; Chung, M.; Kupelnick, B.; Chew, P.; Lau, J. Effects of omega-3 fatty acids on serum markers of cardiovascular disease risk: A systematic review. *Atherosclerosis* **2006**, *189*, 19–30. [CrossRef]
39. Eslick, G.D.; Howe, P.R.C.; Smith, C.; Priest, R.; Bensoussan, A. Benefits of fish oil supplementation in hyperlipidemia: A systematic review and meta-analysis. *Int. J. Cardiol.* **2009**, *136*, 4–16. [CrossRef]
40. Wei, M.Y.; Jacobson, T.A. Effects of eicosapentaenoic acid versus docosahexaenoic acid on serum lipids: A systematic review and meta-analysis. *Curr. Atheroscler. Rep.* **2011**, *13*, 474–483. [CrossRef]
41. DeFilippis, A.P.; Blaha, M.J.; Ndumele, C.E.; Budoff, M.J.; Lloyd-Jones, D.M.; McClelland, R.L.; Lakoski, S.G.; Cushman, M.; Wong, N.D.; Blumenthal, R.S.; et al. The association of Framingham and reynolds risk scores with incidence and progression of coronary artery calcification in MESA (multi-ethnic study of atherosclerosis). *J. Am. Coll. Cardiol.* **2011**, *58*, 2076–2083. [CrossRef]
42. Omar, Z.A.; Montser, B.A.; Farahat, M.A.R. Effect of high-dose Omega 3 on lipid profile and inflammatory markers in chronic hemodialysis children. *Saudi J. Kidney Dis. Transpl.* **2019**, *30*, 634–639. [CrossRef] [PubMed]
43. Miller, M.; Ballantyne, C.M.; Bays, H.E.; Granowitz, C.; Doyle, R.T.; Juliano, R.A.; Philip, S. Effects of Icosapent Ethyl (Eicosapentaenoic Acid Ethyl Ester) on Atherogenic Lipid/Lipoprotein, Apolipoprotein, and Inflammatory Parameters in Patients With Elevated High-Sensitivity C-Reactive Protein (from the ANCHOR Study). *Am. J. Cardiol.* **2019**, *124*, 696–701. [CrossRef] [PubMed]
44. Liew, S.M.; Doust, J.; Glasziou, P. Cardiovascular risk scores do not account for the effect of treatment: A review. *Heart* **2011**, *97*, 689–697. [CrossRef] [PubMed]

Review

Pathobiological Relationship of Excessive Dietary Intake of Choline/L-Carnitine: A TMAO Precursor-Associated Aggravation in Heart Failure in Sarcopenic Patients

May Nasser Bin-Jumah [1,2], Sadaf Jamal Gilani [3], Salman Hosawi [4], Fahad A. Al-Abbasi [4], Mustafa Zeyadi [4], Syed Sarim Imam [5], Sultan Alshehri [5], Mohammed M Ghoneim [6], Muhammad Shahid Nadeem [4] and Imran Kazmi [4,*]

1. Biology Department, College of Science, Princess Nourah Bint Abdulrahman University, Riyadh 11671, Saudi Arabia; mnbinjumah@pnu.edu.sa
2. Environment and Biomaterial Unit, Health Sciences Research Center, Princess Nourah bint Abdulrahman University, Riyadh 11671, Saudi Arabia
3. Department of Basic Health Sciences, Preparatory Year, Princess Nourah Bint Abdulrahman University, Riyadh 11671, Saudi Arabia; SJGlani@pnu.edu.sa
4. Department of Biochemistry, Faculty of Science, King Abdulaziz University, Jeddah 21589, Saudi Arabia; shosawi@kau.edu.sa (S.H.); fabbasi@kau.edu.sa (F.A.A.-A.); mzyadi@kau.edu.sa (M.Z.); mhalim@kau.edu.sa (M.S.N.)
5. Department of Pharmaceutics, College of Pharmacy, King Saud University, Riyadh 11451, Saudi Arabia; simam@ksu.edu.sa (S.S.I.); salshehri1@ksu.edu.sa (S.A.)
6. Department of Pharmacy Practice, College of Pharmacy, AlMaarefa University, Ad Diriyah 13713, Saudi Arabia; mghoneim@mcst.edu.sa
* Correspondence: ikazmi@kau.edu.sa

Abstract: The microecological environment of the gastrointestinal tract is altered if there is an imbalance between the gut microbiota phylases, resulting in a variety of diseases. Moreover, progressive age not only slows down physical activity but also reduces the fat metabolism pathway, which may lead to a reduction in the variety of bacterial strains and bacteroidetes' abundance, promoting firmicutes and proteobacteria growth. As a result, dysbiosis reduces physiological adaptability, boosts inflammatory markers, generates ROS, and induces the destruction of free radical macromolecules, leading to sarcopenia in older patients. Research conducted at various levels indicates that the microbiota of the gut is involved in pathogenesis and can be considered as the causative agent of several cardiovascular diseases. Local and systematic inflammatory reactions are caused in patients with heart failure, as ischemia and edema are caused by splanchnic hypoperfusion and enable both bacterial metabolites and bacteria translocation to enter from an intestinal barrier, which is already weakened, to the blood circulation. Multiple diseases, such as HF, include healthy microbe-derived metabolites. These key findings demonstrate that the gut microbiota modulates the host's metabolism, either specifically or indirectly, by generating multiple metabolites. Currently, the real procedures that are an analogy to the symptoms in cardiac pathologies, such as cardiac mass dysfunctions and modifications, are investigated at a minimum level in older patients. Thus, the purpose of this review is to summarize the existing knowledge about a particular diet, including trimethylamine, which usually seems to be effective for the improvement of cardiac and skeletal muscle, such as choline and L-carnitine, which may aggravate the HF process in sarcopenic patients.

Keywords: sarcopenia; heart failure; trimethylamine-N-oxide; inflammatory mediators; choline; L-carnitine

1. Introduction

The human intestine microbiota is primarily comprised of four phyla: proteobacteria, firmicutes, actinobacteria, and bacteroidetes [1]. An imbalance between the gut microbiota phylases alters the microecological environment of a gastrointestinal tract, resulting in numerous diseases. The gut microbiota has many important functions in sustaining host fitness, including host feeding and energy harvesting, intestinal homeostasis, drug absorption and toxicity, immune system responsiveness, and pathogen defense. They can also produce microbial products such as bile acids, trimethylamine-N-oxide (TMAO), lipopolysaccharides (LPS), vitamin B complexes, vitamin K, uremic toxins, nitric oxide, fatty acids in the short-chain (SCFA), gut neurotransmitters, and hormones, which can modify host metabolism and influence both the health and diseases working in the body [2]. Moreover, progressive age not only slows down physical activity but also reduces the fat metabolism pathway, which may lead to a reduction in the variety of bacterial strains and bacteroidetes' abundance, promoting *firmicutes* and *proteobacteria* growth. As a result, dysbiosis reduces physiological adaptability, boosts inflammatory markers, creates ROS, and induces the destruction of free radical macromolecules, leading to sarcopenia in older patients [3,4]. As aging became a global epidemic, decreased muscle mass in octogenarians (or older persons) impaired 5–13% of elderly people between 60 and 70 years old and has an incidence rate of up to 50% [5]. In a multi-continent sample, sarcopenia prevalence in the general population was between 12.6% and 17.5% [6].

Sarcopenia may be induced by heart failure via common pathogenetic pathways and mechanisms influenced by each other, such as physical activities, malnutrition, and hormonal changes. Prevalence levels are significantly greater in individuals with heart failure (HF), ranging between 19.5 and 47.3% [7].

Conversely, the development of heart failure may be favored by Sarcopenia via various mechanisms such as pathological ergoreflexes. It can be considered as a paradox that the association of sarcopenia is not visible with a sarcopenic cardiac muscle, while non-functional hypertrophy is displayed by cardiac muscles. In addition, cardiac hypertrophy can be considered as the normal mechanism of cardiac adaptation to the conditions of a rise in systemic demand. Cardiac dysfunctions can be caused by a hypertensive state in pregnancy and even in athletes via the heart's physiological hypertrophy or via pathological hypertrophy, which can be triggered by various factors such as hemodynamic stress of irregular and prolonged nature, i.e., a hypertensive condition [4]. Cardiac cachexia has long been shown to be associated with decreased survival and this result can be considered independent of other prognostic variables such as low peak oxygen consumption, age, NYHA (New York Heritage Association) class, or LVEF (left ventricular ejection fraction) [8]. Additionally, research demonstrates a strong link between micronutrients such as Mg^{2+} and cardiovascular health, and highlights the potential pathophysiological pathways through which Mg^{2+} depletion may increase the development, progression, and maintenance of CVD. Indeed, hypomagnesemia has a detrimental effect on cardiovascular health, as it is linked with an increased prevalence of hypertension, type 2 diabetes, dyslipidemia, atherosclerosis, arrhythmias, and coronary artery disease [9], all of which are common in sarcopenia [10].

Enhanced muscle reflex has a significant link with peripheral muscle wastage and, additionally, the overactivity of muscle reflex can be considered consistent with the idea that the development of a syndrome is linked to the muscle's peripheral maladaptive changes. There are some important factors, such as progressive age, associated with sarcopenia and the change in gut microbiota diversity. Dysbiosis can also be considered as an independent cardiovascular risk factor and as responsible for heart failure in elderly people. Minimal investigations have been conducted in elderly patients regarding the actual mechanisms, such as concerning cardiac mass alteration and dysfunction, which are considered equivalent with cardiovascular diseases. They can be concluded as the downward spiral of dysregulation regarding exercise of the skeletal muscle, which is suggested by the hypothesis of muscle and can be correlated with certain vicious cycles in heart failure in which, initially, there are adaptive physiological responses that are gradually converted into maladaptive responses [11]. Thus, the purpose of this review is to summarize the existing knowledge about a particular diet including trimethylamine, which usually seems to be effective for the improvement of cardiac and skeletal muscle, such as choline and L-carnitine, which may aggravate the HF process in sarcopenic patients.

2. Consideration of the Sources for the Review of Literature

Certain databases such as Medline, Mendeley, Google Scholar, Public Library of Science, PubMed, ScienceDirect, and Springer Link were considered and searched through for the literature review, searching for studies that were potentially relevant and in which certain keywords were used both alone and in conjunction. Certain keywords that were significant and were used for the search of literature were 'Sarcopenia', 'Epidemiology of sarcopenia', 'Mechanism of sarcopenia mediated heart failure', 'Involvement of dysbiosis in sarcopenia', 'Pathogenesis of heart failure', 'Reactive oxygen species-mediated mitochondrial dysfunction, 'Relationship of choline and L-carnitine for muscle function improvement' or 'Role of TMA and TMAO in heart failure, in combination with 'heart failure and dysbiosis', 'Immunogenic profile in sarcopenia and heart failure', and 'ergoreflx mechanism in sarcopenia associated heart failure'. In this review, only papers in English were considered. The reference list of the papers found were also screened for related articles not detected by the initial search strategy.

3. Clinical Characteristics of Sarcopenia in Association with Gut Microbiota Diversity

Sarcopenia can be referred to as the gradual loss in mass of skeletal muscle, the loss of its strength, and the loss of functions performed, and it is now considered as the major factor of negative effects of health in the later period of life [12]. In fact, the high pervasiveness of chronic health conditions can be correlated with old age (e.g., inflammatory irritable bowel syndrome, celiac disease, autoimmune disease, colitis, diabetes, cancer, cardiovascular disease, neurodegeneration, and so on), which lead in turn to many negative health events (e.g., illness, loss of freedom, institutionalization, underprivileged quality of life, and mortality) [13–15].

The authors established a link between health status, diet, and microbiota. To be more precise, the composition of the microbial population was predominantly influenced by fruit, meat, and vegetable intake. Additionally, a higher proportion of two dominant phyla, namely Firmicutes (64%) and Bacteroidetes (23%), comprise up to 90% of the overall gut microbiota in older people who are living in long-term care facilities [16–18]). It has been identified that the level of Staphylococcus spp. and Lactobacillus Reuters, both of which are from phylum firmicutes, is high in obese people. A positive correlation has been established between plasma > C-reactive protein (CRP) and plasma [19,20]. Moreover, older people are primarily affected by a rise in Escherichia (phylum of proteobacteria) abundance [16]. However, it is understood that an increase in gram-negative bacteria such as proteobacteria in their relative abundance is one of the most significant harmful age-changes for the human intestinal microbiota composition, as lipopolysaccharides are secreted by these gram-negative bacteria, through which inflammation can be induced in the intestines [21]. Advancing age can also be characterized by a gastrointestinal microbiota's dysbiosis, which promotes the circulation passage of endotoxin and other microbial products or metabolites via the increased permeability of the intestine [22], thereby highlighting the influential role of gut dysbiosis for deficits in muscle functions associated with age. Sarcopenic patients have increased serum c-reactive protein (CRP) levels, while trials with other inflammatory mediators such as interleukin 6 have not shown consistent results [23].

In addition, the maintenance of sarcopenia is supported by the insufficient nutritional system and aged immune system, which play key roles in stimulating the activation of chronic inflammation [24,25]. In cachexia and sarcopenia, however, mitochondrial and systemic inflammation plays a central role. The proinflammatory role of cytokines (e.g., IL6, IL1β, TNF-α, and TNF-style weak apoptosis inducer (TWEAK)) has previously been reported in inducting muscle catabolism [26] (Figure 1).

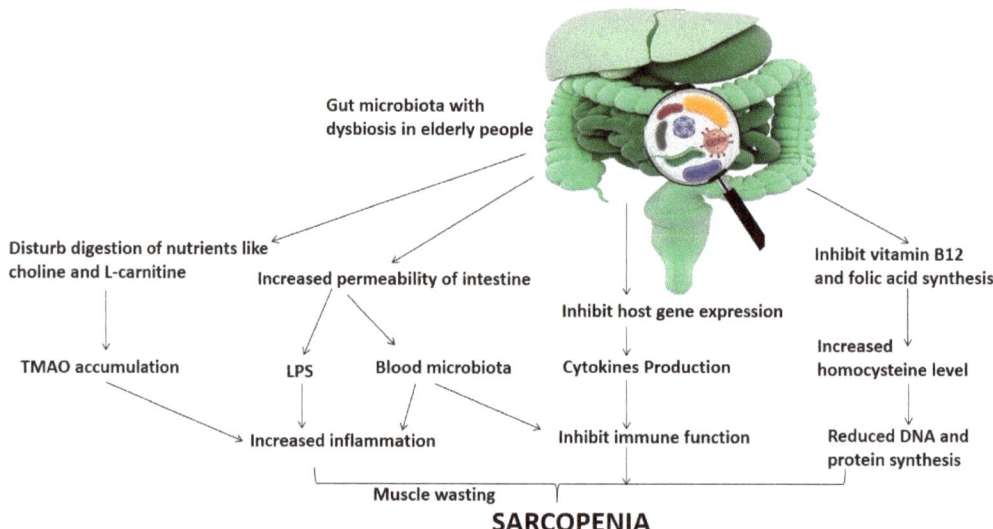

Figure 1. Representation of the relationship of gut microbiota dysbiosis-mediated sarcopenia in elderly people.

4. Dietary Intake Choline and L-Carnitine-Mediated Aggravation of CVD

Choline/L-carnitine was investigated as an ergogenic aid for improving the training ability of a stable athletic population due to its pivotal role in the oxidation of fatty acids and energy metabolism. Beneficial impacts on acute physical performance, such as increased power production and increased intake of maximum oxygen, were observed in earlier research studies and further studies show the beneficial influence of L-carnitine as a dietary supplementation in the post-exercise recovery process. L-carnitine has been shown to alleviate the injury of muscles and condenses' cellular damage markers, and muscle soreness attenuation is accompanied by free radical formation [27].

In 2013, researchers first demonstrated that a molecular metabolite, namely trimethylamine-N-oxide (TMAO) isolated from the microbiota of the gut, predicted that 4007 healthy cardiac patients will be enduring elective coronary angiography with an excepted increased risk of cardiovascular accidents [28]. TMAO is produced by microbiota via the ingestion of meat products containing nutritional precursors of trimethylamine, such as phosphatidylcholine, glycerophosphocholine, trimethylglycine, betaine, γ-butyrobetaine, crotonobetaine, choline, and L-carnitine [28–31]. Specific intestinal microbial enzymes convert these precursors into trimethylamine and to date, they have identified four different types of microbial enzyme systems including choline-TMA lyase (cutC/D) [32], carnitine monooxygenase (cntA/B) [33], betaine reductase [34], and TMAO reductase [35]. Recently, it has also been demonstrated that elevated L-carnitine, choline, and phosphatidylcholine amounts reflect multiple cardiovascular hazards such as myocardial infarction, hypertension, atherosclerosis, and diabetes [36–43].

Change in the microbiota composition of the gut caused by sarcopenia and heart failure can alter the circulating levels of TMAO. Moreover, it has been identified that hypertension patients experience an alteration in intestinal microbiota diversity. Experiments conducted on rats who were treated with angiotensin II revealed that intestinal biota species were less diverse and when compared to regulated rats, the Firmicutes to Bacteroidetes ratio was increased [44,45]. Moreover, heart failure was considered a chronic systemic inflammatory disorder, which indicates a substantial rise in pro-inflammatory cytokines of plasma; although its origin is still unclear, this unresolved inflammation can be considered as one of the key components of cardiovascular diseases [46,47]. Several occurring signs indicate that the microbiota of the gut produces bioactive metabolites including bile acids, short chains of fatty acids, and TMAO, and might have systemic effects on the host [48]. Microbiotas and their metabolites affect intestinal health and other physiological processes, especially within the circulatory system. Under normal circumstances, most can be considered as healthy and safe bacterial metabolites, but due to the involvement of heart-failure-related cardiovascular pathologic processes, there is a risk of disruption in the balance of the microbiota of the gut as well as a risk of a rise in the level of harmful metabolites; generally, it was shown in studies that TMAO was found to be related with the prognosis of at-risk heart-failure patients. Moreover, Firmicutes, including Enterococcus, Proteobacteria, Anaerococcus, Streptococcus, and Desulfitobacterium including Actinobacteria, Clostridium, Citrobacter, Dseulfovibrio Enterobacter, Escherichia, Proteus, Pseudomonas, and Klebsiella, have been linked with the production of the primary component of TMAO, i.e., TMA [49].

One research study found that eight Firmicute and Proteobacteria species have absorbed more than 60% of the production of choline of TMA, including Escherichia fergusonii, Clostridium asparagiforme, C. hathawayi, C. sporogenes, Edwardsiella tarda Anaerococcus hydrogenalis, Proteus penneri, and Providencia rettgeri [50]. Akkermansia, Prevotella, and Sporobacter are some other gut microbiota that are associated with the higher production of TMAO [51], and atherosclerotic CAD is associated with Ruminococcus gnavus [52]. The growth of CAD may be predicted via different metabolites such as betaine, choline, and TMA. It can be explained, for instance, by considering that TMAO-producing microbes can be reduced by blocking or inhibiting specific microbial metabolic pathways via utilizing pharmacological intervention and probiotics [53]. Furthermore, the increased level of *Ruminococcus* is due to the high fat and high protein diet [54], and additionally, downregulation of Treg cells is led by TLR4 activation, which is associated with inflammatory responses such as CD4, Pro-inflammatory cytokines, and Th1 and T cells [55,56]. Thus, we explore, from top to bottom, all of the contributing factors associated with CVD.

5. Pathobiological Interactions in Heart Failure Involving TMAO

Mechanisms of heart failure pathophysiological pathways are quite intricate and include inflammatory reaction, hemodynamics irregularity, cardiac remodeling, neuroendocrine system stimulation, etc. Traditionally, the key causes of heart failure are supposed to be the activation of the pathways of the neuroendocrine system, which include the natriuretic peptide system, renin-angiotensin-aldosterone cascade, and sympathetic nervous system, which lead to a pathologic myocardial remodeling process series including apoptosis, extracellular matrix deposition, myocardial hypertrophy, and resultant fibrosis [57,58]. Hence, neuroendocrine inhibition is the main basis of the strategies of current treatments [59]. Mechanisms driving the development and progression of heart failure are, however, still under consideration. In the conversion of dietary choline into the intermediate trimethylamine (TMA), a requisite role is played by microbiota of the gut and TMAO is formed by the subsequent oxidization of TMA after it enters into the circulatory system by the flavin-containing monooxygenase (FMO) enzyme, which is encoded by the FMO gene present in the kidney, liver, and in many other tissues [60,61]. There is an increase in the permeability of the intestinal barrier via two mechanisms in the condition of heart failure, in which during the initial stage, a decreased inflow of blood to the intestinal endothelium is observed, and via the ischemia of the wall of the intestine, there is an increase in the permeability of the intestinal epithelial barrier [62]. Due to the intestinal wall's congestion and swelling in the advanced stages of heart failure, there is an increase in the permeability of the intestine. Additionally, in the patients identified with chronic heart failure, higher levels of enteropathogenic candida, such as Campylobacter, Shigella, and Salmonella, were observed [63]. This process is directly linked with microbial and microbial metabolite translocation [64,65]. Recent research evidence indicates that chronic inflammation can be caused by both an increase in the permeability and an increase in the disordered microbiota of the intestine, further leading to impaired cardiac function [62,66]. In addition, studies have shown that there are severe clinical symptoms and worse survival rates associated with patients with heart failure, which are due to the elevated serum levels of multiple cytokines, such as IL-1, IL-6, and the TNF [67–69]. This is consistent with findings that both heart failure and sarcopenic patients have an elevated proportion of these bacterial strains of the intestine, indicating shifts in intestinal microbiota, which may influence levels of TMAO by controlling intestinal TMA synthesis. TMAO has recently become a major mediator showing that the microbiota of the gut has a close relationship with several CVDs. Subsequent preclinical experiments explored the evidence concerning that the heart is directly affected by the TMAO, inducing endothelial cell and vascular inflammation, fibrosis and myocardial hypertrophy, and heart mitochondrial dysfunction, thus aggravating the heart-failure process [70–72]. In addition, the association of TMAO is established with both the C-reactive protein (CRP) and with endothelial dysfunction in evaluating the increased permeability of the gut, and is closely related to increased LPS endotoxin serum levels [49], leading to the release of calcium and the hyperreactivity of the platelets [73], contributing to the aggravation of heart failure. The several key pathophysiological pathways of TMAO include the following: explicitly and implicitly contributing in heart failure, including through the pathological LV dilation of the mouse-fed TMAO or choline-demonstrated decreased LVEF, and enhanced circulatory BNP volumes, myocardial fibrosis, and lung oedema [31]; TMAO-encouraged myocardial hypertrophy and fibrosis through Smad3 signals [71]; cardiac remodeling attenuated through 3,3-dimethyl-1-butanol via the reduction in the volume of plasma TMAO, which modifies the signals of TGF-β1/Smad3 and p65 NF-kB [74]; TMAO-promoted activated leukocyte recruitment into endothelial cells and induced inflammatory gene expression via the activation of NF-kB signaling [75]; TMAO significantly affected the contractile nature of cardiomyocyte and intracellular calcium-handling in the negative direction [76]; Pyruvates and fatty acid oxidation in cardiac mitochondria is influenced by TMAO [70]; and, last but not least, TMAO stimulated vascular inflammation by triggering the inflammatory NLRP3 induced by inhibiting SIRT3-SOD2–mitochondrial ROS signaling pathway [77]. Moreover, the function of TMAO, as first assessed by Suzuki et al. [78] in acute HF (AHF), was found to be a predicting marker for mortality and mortality/heart failure within a year (Table 1) [79].

Table 1. TMA metabolism-targeting therapeutic methods.

Therapy	Alteration in Biotransformation TMA	Implications
Inhibition of the FMO3 enzyme	Prevents oxidation of TMA to TMAO	Trimethylaminuria is caused by an accumulation of TMA and is characterized by a fishy odor. It may also cause inflammation. Additionally, FMO3 metabolizes a wide variety of other compounds.
Resveratrol	Modifies the makeup of the gut microbiota. Reduces the formation of TMA and TMAO.	Increases *Lactobacillus* and *Bifidobacterium*. When antibiotics are taken, no adverse effects occur. Observed in mice studies.
Enalapril	Increases TMAO excretion in the urine	Mechanism unknown. Rat studies were conducted. It does not affect TMA synthesis or the makeup of the gut flora.
Prebiotics	Induces a beneficial effect on the makeup of the gut bacteria to reduce TMA production in the intestine	In humans, the consequences are unknown. Numerous variables affect the makeup of the gut microbiota.
Probiotics (I): Methanogenic bacteria	Reduces TMA and TMAO levels	Human safety and engraftment are unknown.
Probiotics (II): Bacteria incapable of converting precursors to TMA	Reduces the production of TMA in the gut	Mice show beneficial benefits. However, the consequences on people remain unknown.

Table 1. *Cont.*

Therapy	Alteration in Biotransformation TMA	Implications
Meldonium	Reduces the production of TMAO from L-carnitine (GBB conversion to L-carnitine is inhibited)	TMAO production from choline cannot be reduced. It may result in a rise in the urine excretion of TMAO in people.
Oral non-absorbent binders	Eliminates TMAO or any of its precursors from the gut	A speculative approach. There has not yet been found a chemical capable of removing TMAO specifically.

Additionally, an independent cohort of ambulatory individuals with persistent systolic HF supports our results and provides new insights on the link between the three phosphatidylcholine metabolic isomers, namely TMAO, choline, and betaine, considering echocardiographic determinants and the associations between both renal and inflammatory biomarkers. Numerous noteworthy discoveries have been made. To begin, we found that TMAO had a superior predictive value to choline and betaine in patients with chronic systolic heart failure, regardless of the cardio-renal parameters. Second, rather than LV systolic dysfunction, we found associations between all three metabolites and LV diastolic dysfunction. Thirdly, the very low correlations between TMAO, choline, and betaine in many well-characterized inflammatory biomarkers and in their distinct associations with endothelial dysfunction indicators indicated the existence of a separate pathophysiological mechanism. Notably, the increased TMAO levels seen in individuals with renal insufficiency or diabetes mellitus suggest an underlying metabolic deficiency associated with those disease states rather than a systemic inflammatory response. Nonetheless, the relationship between increased TMAO and both HF severity and adverse outcomes, irrespective of other cardio-renal indices, argues for a possible harmful molecular link between the gut microbiota pathway that generates TMAO and the development and/or progression of HF. Notably, this is a cohort of ambulatory stable heart failure patients with left ventricular systolic dysfunction and with an annualized mortality of 7.1% (considering transplantation as the equivalent of death), which is not dissimilar to that seen in published clinical trials. Taken together, our results validate the clinical relevance of TMAO levels in heart failure and indicate that further research is needed to elucidate the association's molecular underpinnings. However, after tuning for the parameters of renal function, the capacity of the TMAO to independently forecast is lost, likely due to the substantial correlations between the parameters of renal function (approximate glomerular filtration rate and urea) and TMAO. These findings indicate that a higher degree of "backward failure" (congestion associated with scarring or ischemia) rather than "forward failure" (or reduced perfusion) may be linked with the main metabolic deficiency underlying the observed correlations. Consistent with this, correlations between choline and renal function indices were seen for both choline and TMAO, although the link between TMAO and adverse outcomes in individuals persisted even after adjusting for renal function. The purpose of this study was to investigate the connection between (1) the intestinal microbiota-dependent analyte TMAO and its dietary precursors, namely and choline and betaine, and (2) echocardiographic indicators in sarcopenic patients with chronic systolic heart failure [80,81] (Figure 2).

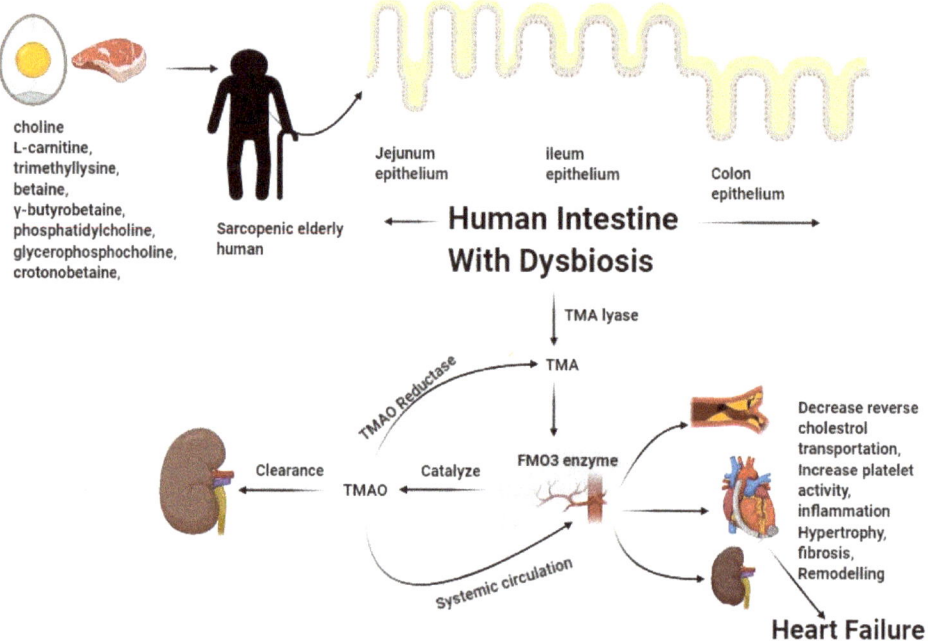

Figure 2. Representation demonstrating the pathobiological relationship of the excessive intake of choline/L-carnitine-containing diet-associated TMAO accumulation, resulting in the heart failure of sarcopenic patients.

6. Conclusions

Sarcopenia is common in cases of heart failure, leading to inadequate disease prognosis. While the pathophysiology of muscle wastage is quite complicated in heart failure, multiple pathogenetic mechanisms tend to be shared by sarcopenia and heart failure, and they can benefit from strategies of standard treatment focused on a nutritional, physical, and pharmacological approach. In recent years, several studies have identified a clear correlation between CVDs and the microbiota of the gut. We already know that TMAO, a gut microbiota metabolite, may have fresh perspectives and insights regarding how heart failure is supported by the microbiota of the gut. These findings provide a good opportunity for controlling heart failure via addressing the microbiota of the gut, including through the use of updated probiotics, prebiotics, dietary therapy, and FMT. Moreover, emerging research from different groups and clinical findings reveal the association between the dysfunction of the microbiota of the gut, the TMAO circulation, and the susceptibility of heart failure, indicating a fresh and desirable therapeutic target for HF treatment. Furthermore, excessive intake of a diet such as choline or L-carnitine, which contain intermediate precursor TMA for TMAO, should be carefully used in elderly people who have dysbiosis with muscle disorders. Future research studies are warranted.

Author Contributions: Conceptualization and methodology, I.K. and M.N.B.-J.; writing—original draft preparation, S.J.G., S.H., F.A.A.-A. and I.K.; writing—review and editing, S.S.I., M.Z. and M.S.N.; supervision, S.A. and M.M.G.; project administration, I.K. All authors have read and agreed to the published version of the manuscript.

Funding: This research received no external funding.

Acknowledgments: Authors are thankful for Deanship of Library Affairs, King Abdulaziz University for providing online access of articles.

Conflicts of Interest: The authors declare no conflict of interest.

References

1. Wu, G.D.; Bushmanc, F.D.; Lewis, J.D. Diet, the human gut microbiota, and IBD. *Anaerobe* **2013**, *24*, 117–120. [CrossRef]
2. Kazemian, N.; Mahmoudi, M.; Halperin, F.; Wu, J.C.; Pakpour, S. Gut microbiota and cardiovascular disease: Opportunities and challenges. *Microbiome* **2020**, *8*, 36. [CrossRef]
3. Wu, G.D.; Chen, J.; Hoffmann, C.; Bittinger, K.; Chen, Y.Y.; Keilbaugh, S.A.; Bewtra, M.; Knights, D.; Walters, W.A.; Knight, R.; et al. Linking long-term dietary patterns with gut microbial enterotypes. *Science* **2011**, *334*, 105–108. [CrossRef] [PubMed]
4. Shimizu, I.; Minamino, T. Physiological and pathological cardiac hypertrophy. *J. Mol. Cell. Cardiol.* **2016**, *97*, 245–262. [CrossRef] [PubMed]
5. von Haehling, S.; Morley, J.E.; Anker, S.D. An overview of sarcopenia: Facts and numbers on prevalence and clinical impact. *J. Cachexia Sarcopenia Muscle* **2010**, *1*, 129–133. [CrossRef] [PubMed]
6. Tyrovolas, S.; Koyanagi, A.; Olaya, B.; Ayuso-Mateos, J.L.; Miret, M.; Chatterji, S.; Tobiasz-Adamczyk, B.; Koskinen, S.; Leonardi, M.; Haro, J.M. Factors associated with skeletal muscle mass, sarcopenia, and sarcopenic obesity in older adults: A multi-continent study. *J. Cachexia Sarcopenia Muscle* **2016**, *7*, 312–321. [CrossRef]
7. Hajahmadi, M.; Shemshadi, S.; Khalilipur, E.; Amin, A.; Taghavi, S.; Maleki, M.; Malek, H.; Naderi, N. Muscle wasting in young patients with dilated cardiomyopathy. *J. Cachexia Sarcopenia Muscle* **2017**, *8*, 542–548. [CrossRef]
8. Anker, S.D.; Ponikowski, P.; Varney, S.; Chua, T.P.; Clark, A.L.; Webb-Peploe, K.M.; Harrington, D.; Kox, W.J.; Poole-Wilson, P.A.; Coats, A.J. Wasting as independent risk factor for mortality in chronic heart failure. *Lancet* **1997**, *349*, 1050–1053. [CrossRef]
9. Severino, P.; Netti, L.; Mariani, M.V.; Maraone, A.; D'Amato, A.; Scarpati, R.; Infusino, F.; Pucci, M.; Lavalle, C.; Maestrini, C.; et al. Prevention of Cardiovascular Disease: Screening for Magnesium Deficiency. *Cardiol. Res. Pract.* **2019**, *2019*, 4874921. [CrossRef] [PubMed]
10. Dominguez, L.J.; Barbagallo, M.; Lauretani, F.; Bandinelli, S.; Bos, A.; Corsi, A.M.; Simonsick, E.M.; Ferrucci, L. Magnesium and muscle performance in older persons: The InCHIANTI study. *Am. J. Clin. Nutr.* **2006**, *84*, 419–426. [CrossRef] [PubMed]
11. Piepoli, M.F.; Kaczmarek, A.; Francis, D.P.; Davies, L.C.; Rauchhaus, M.; Jankowska, E.A.; Anker, S.D.; Capucci, A.; Banasiak, W.; Ponikowski, P. Reduced Peripheral Skeletal Muscle Mass and Abnormal Reflex Physiology in Chronic Heart Failure. *Circulation* **2006**, *114*, 126–134. [CrossRef] [PubMed]
12. Marzetti, E.; Calvani, R.; Tosato, M.; Cesari, M.; Di Bari, M.; Cherubini, A.; Collamati, A.; D'Angelo, E.; Pahor, M.; Bernabei, R.; et al. Sarcopenia: An overview. *Aging Clin. Exp. Res.* **2017**, *29*, 11–17. [CrossRef] [PubMed]
13. Cesari, M.; Marzetti, E.; Thiem, U.; Pérez-Zepeda, M.U.; Abellan Van Kan, G.; Landi, F.; Petrovic, M.; Cherubini, A.; Bernabei, R. The geriatric management of frailty as paradigm of "The end of the disease era". *Eur. J. Intern. Med.* **2016**, *31*, 11–14. [CrossRef] [PubMed]
14. Arumugam, M.; Raes, J.; Pelletier, E.; Le Paslier, D.; Yamada, T.; Mende, D.R.; Fernandes, G.R.; Tap, J.; Bruls, T.; Batto, J.M.; et al. Enterotypes of the human gut microbiome. *Nature* **2011**, *473*, 174–180. [CrossRef] [PubMed]
15. Saraswati, S.; Sitaraman, R. Aging and the human gut microbiota—from correlation to causality. *Front. Microbiol.* **2015**, *5*, 764. [CrossRef]
16. Claesson, M.J.; Jeffery, I.B.; Conde, S.; Power, S.E.; O'Connor, E.M.; Cusack, S.; Harris, H.M.; Coakley, M.; Lakshminarayanan, B.; O'Sullivan, O.; et al. Gut microbiota composition correlates with diet and health in the elderly. *Nature* **2012**, *488*, 178–184. [CrossRef] [PubMed]
17. Huttenhower, C.; Gevers, D.; Knight, R.; Abubucker, S.; Badger, J.H.; Chinwalla, A.T.; Creasy, H.H.; Earl, A.M.; FitzGerald, M.G.; Fulton, R.S.; et al. Structure, function and diversity of the healthy human microbiome. *Nature* **2012**, *486*, 207–214. [CrossRef]
18. Dethlefsen, L.; McFall-Ngai, M.; Relman, D.A. An ecological and evolutionary perspective on human-microbe mutualism and disease. *Nature* **2007**, *449*, 811–818. [CrossRef] [PubMed]
19. Bervoets, L.; Van Hoorenbeeck, K.; Kortleven, I.; Van Noten, C.; Hens, N.; Vael, C.; Goossens, H.; Desager, K.N.; Vankerckhoven, V. Differences in gut microbiota composition between obese and lean children: A cross-sectional study. *Gut Pathog.* **2013**, *5*, 10. [CrossRef]
20. Million, M.; Angelakis, E.; Paul, M.; Armougom, F.; Leibovici, L.; Raoult, D. Comparative meta-analysis of the effect of *Lactobacillus* species on weight gain in humans and animals. *Microb. Pathog.* **2012**, *53*, 100–108. [CrossRef]
21. Kumar, M.; Babaei, P.; Ji, B.; Nielsen, J. Human gut microbiota and healthy aging: Recent developments and future prospective. *Nutr. Healthy Aging* **2016**, *4*, 3–16. [CrossRef] [PubMed]
22. Pitchumoni, C.; Mishra, S.P.; Yadav, H. Gut Microbiota and Aging: A Broad Perspective. In *Geriatric Gastroenterology*; Pitchumoni, C.S., Dharmarajan, T.S., Eds.; Springer International Publishing: Cham, Switzerland, 2020; pp. 1–21. [CrossRef]
23. Bano, G.; Trevisan, C.; Carraro, S.; Solmi, M.; Luchini, C.; Stubbs, B.; Manzato, E.; Sergi, G.; Veronese, N. Inflammation and sarcopenia: A systematic review and meta-analysis. *Maturitas* **2017**, *96*, 10–15. [CrossRef] [PubMed]
24. Ticinesi, A.; Meschi, T.; Lauretani, F.; Felis, G.; Franchi, F.; Pedrolli, C.; Barichella, M.; Benati, G.; Di Nuzzo, S.; Ceda, G.P.; et al. Nutrition and Inflammation in Older Individuals: Focus on Vitamin D, n-3 Polyunsaturated Fatty Acids and Whey Proteins. *Nutrients* **2016**, *8*, 186. [CrossRef] [PubMed]
25. Wilson, D.; Jackson, T.; Sapey, E.; Lord, J.M. Frailty and sarcopenia: The potential role of an aged immune system. *Ageing Res. Rev.* **2017**, *36*, 1–10. [CrossRef]

26. Zhou, J.; Liu, B.; Liang, C.; Li, Y.; Song, Y.H. Cytokine Signaling in Skeletal Muscle Wasting. *Trends Endocrinol. Metab. TEM* **2016**, *27*, 335–347. [CrossRef] [PubMed]
27. Fielding, R.; Riede, L.; Lugo, J.P.; Bellamine, A. l-Carnitine Supplementation in Recovery after Exercise. *Nutrients* **2018**, *10*, 349. [CrossRef] [PubMed]
28. Wang, Z.; Klipfell, E.; Bennett, B.J.; Koeth, R.; Levison, B.S.; Dugar, B.; Feldstein, A.E.; Britt, E.B.; Fu, X.; Chung, Y.M.; et al. Gut flora metabolism of phosphatidylcholine promotes cardiovascular disease. *Nature* **2011**, *472*, 57–63. [CrossRef]
29. Tang, W.H.; Hazen, S.L. The contributory role of gut microbiota in cardiovascular disease. *J. Clin. Investig.* **2014**, *124*, 4204–4211. [CrossRef]
30. Wang, Z.; Zhao, Y. Gut microbiota derived metabolites in cardiovascular health and disease. *Protein Cell.* **2018**, *9*, 416–431. [CrossRef]
31. Organ, C.L.; Otsuka, H.; Bhushan, S.; Wang, Z.; Bradley, J.; Trivedi, R.; Polhemus, D.J.; Tang, W.H.; Wu, Y.; Hazen, S.L.; et al. Choline Diet and Its Gut Microbe-Derived Metabolite, Trimethylamine N-Oxide, Exacerbate Pressure Overload-Induced Heart Failure. *Circ. Heart Fail.* **2016**, *9*, e002314. [CrossRef]
32. Craciun, S.; Marks, J.A.; Balskus, E.P. Characterization of choline trimethylamine-lyase expands the chemistry of glycyl radical enzymes. *ACS Chem. Biol.* **2014**, *9*, 1408–1413. [CrossRef] [PubMed]
33. Zhu, Y.; Jameson, E.; Crosatti, M.; Schäfer, H.; Rajakumar, K.; Bugg, T.D.; Chen, Y. Carnitine metabolism to trimethylamine by an unusual Rieske-type oxygenase from human microbiota. *Proc. Natl. Acad. Sci. USA* **2014**, *111*, 4268–4273. [CrossRef]
34. Andreesen, J.R. Glycine metabolism in anaerobes. *Antonie Van Leeuwenhoek* **1994**, *66*, 223–237. [CrossRef] [PubMed]
35. Pascal, M.C.; Burini, J.F.; Chippaux, M. Regulation of the trimethylamine N-oxide (TMAO) reductase in Escherichia coli: Analysis of tor::Mud1 operon fusion. *Mol. Gen. Genet. MGG* **1984**, *195*, 351–355. [CrossRef] [PubMed]
36. Yang, Q.; Liang, Q.; Balakrishnan, B.; Belobrajdic, D.P.; Feng, Q.J.; Zhang, W. Role of Dietary Nutrients in the Modulation of Gut Microbiota: A Narrative Review. *Nutrients* **2020**, *12*, 381. [CrossRef] [PubMed]
37. Rowland, I.; Gibson, G.; Heinken, A.; Scott, K.; Swann, J.; Thiele, I.; Tuohy, K. Gut microbiota functions: Metabolism of nutrients and other food components. *Eur. J. Nutr.* **2018**, *57*, 1–24. [CrossRef] [PubMed]
38. Tang, W.H.; Wang, Z.; Levison, B.S.; Koeth, R.A.; Britt, E.B.; Fu, X.; Wu, Y.; Hazen, S.L. Intestinal microbial metabolism of phosphatidylcholine and cardiovascular risk. *N. Engl. J. Med.* **2013**, *368*, 1575–1584. [CrossRef]
39. Senthong, V.; Wang, Z.; Fan, Y.; Wu, Y.; Hazen, S.L.; Tang, W.H.W. Trimethylamine *N-oxide* and mortality risk in patients with peripheral artery disease. *J. Am. Heart Assoc.* **2016**, *5*, e004237. [CrossRef]
40. Ge, X.; Zheng, L.; Zhuang, R.; Yu, P.; Xu, Z.; Liu, G.; Xi, X.; Zhou, X.; Fan, H. The Gut Microbial Metabolite Trimethylamine N-Oxide and Hypertension Risk: A Systematic Review and Dose-Response Meta-analysis. *Adv. Nutr.* **2020**, *11*, 66–76. [CrossRef]
41. Tan, Y.; Sheng, Z.; Zhou, P.; Liu, C.; Zhao, H.; Song, L.; Li, J.; Zhou, J.; Chen, Y.; Wang, L.; et al. Plasma Trimethylamine N-Oxide as a Novel Biomarker for Plaque Rupture in Patients With ST-Segment-Elevation Myocardial Infarction. *Circ. Cardiovasc. Interv.* **2019**, *12*, e007281. [CrossRef]
42. Ivashkin, V.T.; Kashukh, Y.A. Impact of L-carnitine and phosphatidylcholine containing products on the proatherogenic metabolite TMAO production and gut microbiome changes in patients with coronary artery disease. *Vopr. Pitan.* **2019**, *88*, 25–33. [CrossRef] [PubMed]
43. Tang, W.H.; Wang, Z.; Li, X.S.; Fan, Y.; Li, D.S.; Wu, Y.; Hazen, S.L. Increased Trimethylamine N-Oxide Portends High Mortality Risk Independent of Glycemic Control in Patients with Type 2 Diabetes Mellitus. *Clin. Chem.* **2017**, *63*, 297–306. [CrossRef] [PubMed]
44. Ramezani, A.; Raj, D.S. The gut microbiome, kidney disease, and targeted interventions. *J. Am. Soc. Nephrol. JASN* **2014**, *25*, 657–670. [CrossRef]
45. Pluznick, J.L.; Protzko, R.J.; Gevorgyan, H.; Peterlin, Z.; Sipos, A.; Han, J.; Brunet, I.; Wan, L.X.; Rey, F.; Wang, T.; et al. Olfactory receptor responding to gut microbiota-derived signals plays a role in renin secretion and blood pressure regulation. *Proc. Natl. Acad. Sci. USA* **2013**, *110*, 4410–4415. [CrossRef] [PubMed]
46. Liljestrand, J.M.; Paju, S.; Pietiäinen, M.; Buhlin, K.; Persson, G.R.; Nieminen, M.S.; Sinisalo, J.; Mäntylä, P.; Pussinen, P.J. Immunologic burden links periodontitis to acute coronary syndrome. *Atherosclerosis* **2018**, *268*, 177–184. [CrossRef]
47. Pullen, A.B.; Jadapalli, J.K.; Rhourri-Frih, B.; Halade, G.V. Re-evaluating the causes and consequences of non-resolving inflammation in chronic cardiovascular disease. *Heart Fail. Rev.* **2020**, *25*, 381–391. [CrossRef]
48. Tang, W.H.W.; Li, D.Y.; Hazen, S.L. Dietary metabolism, the gut microbiome, and heart failure. *Nat. Rev. Cardiol.* **2019**, *16*, 137–154. [CrossRef] [PubMed]
49. Al-Obaide, M.A.I.; Singh, R.; Datta, P.; Rewers-Felkins, K.A.; Salguero, M.V.; Al-Obaidi, I.; Kottapalli, K.R.; Vasylyeva, T.L. Gut Microbiota-Dependent Trimethylamine-N-oxide and Serum Biomarkers in Patients with T2DM and Advanced CKD. *J. Clin. Med.* **2017**, *6*, 86. [CrossRef] [PubMed]
50. Liu, T.-X.; Niu, H.-T.; Zhang, S.-Y. Intestinal Microbiota Metabolism and Atherosclerosis. *Chin. Med. J.* **2015**, *128*, 2805–2811. [CrossRef] [PubMed]
51. Falony, G.; Vieira-Silva, S.; Raes, J. Microbiology Meets Big Data: The Case of Gut Microbiota-Derived Trimethylamine. *Annu. Rev. Microbiol.* **2015**, *69*, 305–321. [CrossRef]

52. Wang, Z.; Roberts, A.B.; Buffa, J.A.; Levison, B.S.; Zhu, W.; Org, E.; Gu, X.; Huang, Y.; Zamanian-Daryoush, M.; Culley, M.K.; et al. Non-lethal Inhibition of Gut Microbial Trimethylamine Production for the Treatment of Atherosclerosis. *Cell* **2015**, *163*, 1585–1595. [CrossRef]
53. Martin, F.P.; Wang, Y.; Sprenger, N.; Yap, I.K.; Lundstedt, T.; Lek, P.; Rezzi, S.; Ramadan, Z.; van Bladeren, P.; Fay, L.B.; et al. Probiotic modulation of symbiotic gut microbial-host metabolic interactions in a humanized microbiome mouse model. *Mol. Syst. Biol.* **2008**, *4*, 157. [CrossRef]
54. Kim, K.A.; Gu, W.; Lee, I.A.; Joh, E.H.; Kim, D.H. High fat diet-induced gut microbiota exacerbates inflammation and obesity in mice via the TLR4 signaling pathway. *PLoS ONE* **2012**, *7*, e47713. [CrossRef]
55. Feuerer, M.; Herrero, L.; Cipolletta, D.; Naaz, A.; Wong, J.; Nayer, A.; Lee, J.; Goldfine, A.B.; Benoist, C.; Shoelson, S.; et al. Lean, but not obese, fat is enriched for a unique population of regulatory T cells that affect metabolic parameters. *Nat. Med.* **2009**, *15*, 930–939. [CrossRef]
56. Ilan, Y.; Maron, R.; Tukpah, A.M.; Maioli, T.U.; Murugaiyan, G.; Yang, K.; Wu, H.Y.; Weiner, H.L. Induction of regulatory T cells decreases adipose inflammation and alleviates insulin resistance in ob/ob mice. *Proc. Natl. Acad. Sci. USA* **2010**, *107*, 9765–9770. [CrossRef]
57. Mudd, J.O.; Kass, D.A. Tackling heart failure in the twenty-first century. *Nature* **2008**, *451*, 919–928. [CrossRef]
58. Shah, A.M.; Mann, D.L. In search of new therapeutic targets and strategies for heart failure: Recent advances in basic science. *Lancet* **2011**, *378*, 704–712. [CrossRef]
59. Ponikowski, P.; Voors, A.A.; Anker, S.D.; Bueno, H.; Cleland, J.G.F.; Coats, A.J.S.; Falk, V.; González-Juanatey, J.R.; Harjola, V.P.; Jankowska, E.A.; et al. 2016 ESC Guidelines for the Diagnosis and Treatment of Acute and Chronic Heart Failure. *Rev. Esp. Cardiol.* **2016**, *69*, 1167. [CrossRef] [PubMed]
60. Hernandez, D.; Janmohamed, A.; Chandan, P.; Phillips, I.R.; Shephard, E.A. Organization and evolution of the flavin-containing monooxygenase genes of human and mouse: Identification of novel gene and pseudogene clusters. *Pharmacogenetics* **2004**, *14*, 117–130. [CrossRef] [PubMed]
61. Phillips, I.R.; Dolphin, C.T.; Clair, P.; Hadley, M.R.; Hutt, A.J.; McCombie, R.R.; Smith, R.L.; Shephard, E.A. The molecular biology of the flavin-containing monooxygenases of man. *Chem.-Biol. Interact.* **1995**, *96*, 17–32. [CrossRef]
62. Sandek, A.; Bauditz, J.; Swidsinski, A.; Buhner, S.; Weber-Eibel, J.; von Haehling, S.; Schroedl, W.; Karhausen, T.; Doehner, W.; Rauchhaus, M.; et al. Altered intestinal function in patients with chronic heart failure. *J. Am. Coll. Cardiol.* **2007**, *50*, 1561–1569. [CrossRef]
63. Pasini, E.; Aquilani, R.; Testa, C.; Baiardi, P.; Angioletti, S.; Boschi, F.; Verri, M.; Dioguardi, F. Pathogenic Gut Flora in Patients with Chronic Heart Failure. *JACC. Heart Fail.* **2016**, *4*, 220–227. [CrossRef]
64. Bordalo Tonucci, L.; Dos Santos, K.M.; De Luces Fortes Ferreira, C.L.; Ribeiro, S.M.; De Oliveira, L.L.; Martino, H.S. Gut microbiota and probiotics: Focus on diabetes mellitus. *Crit. Rev. Food Sci. Nutr.* **2017**, *57*, 2296–2309. [CrossRef] [PubMed]
65. Wang, F.; Jiang, H.; Shi, K.; Ren, Y.; Zhang, P.; Cheng, S. Gut bacterial translocation is associated with microinflammation in end-stage renal disease patients. *Nephrology* **2012**, *17*, 733–738. [CrossRef]
66. Cox, A.J.; West, N.P.; Cripps, A.W. Obesity, inflammation, and the gut microbiota. *Lancet Diabetes Endocrinol.* **2015**, *3*, 207–215. [CrossRef]
67. Conraads, V.M.; Bosmans, J.M.; Schuerwegh, A.J.; Goovaerts, I.; De Clerck, L.S.; Stevens, W.J.; Bridts, C.H.; Vrints, C.J. Intracellular monocyte cytokine production and CD 14 expression are up-regulated in severe vs mild chronic heart failure. *J. Heart Lung Transplant. Off. Publ. Int. Soc. Heart Transplant.* **2005**, *24*, 854–859. [CrossRef] [PubMed]
68. Rauchhaus, M.; Doehner, W.; Francis, D.P.; Davos, C.; Kemp, M.; Liebenthal, C.; Niebauer, J.; Hooper, J.; Volk, H.D.; Coats, A.J.; et al. Plasma cytokine parameters and mortality in patients with chronic heart failure. *Circulation* **2000**, *102*, 3060–3067. [CrossRef]
69. Deswal, A.; Petersen, N.J.; Feldman, A.M.; Young, J.B.; White, B.G.; Mann, D.L. Cytokines and cytokine receptors in advanced heart failure: An analysis of the cytokine database from the Vesnarinone trial (VEST). *Circulation* **2001**, *103*, 2055–2059. [CrossRef] [PubMed]
70. Makrecka-Kuka, M.; Volska, K.; Antone, U.; Vilskersts, R.; Grinberga, S.; Bandere, D.; Liepinsh, E.; Dambrova, M. Trimethylamine N-oxide impairs pyruvate and fatty acid oxidation in cardiac mitochondria. *Toxicol. Lett.* **2017**, *267*, 32–38. [CrossRef] [PubMed]
71. Li, Z.; Wu, Z.; Yan, J.; Liu, H.; Liu, Q.; Deng, Y.; Ou, C.; Chen, M. Gut microbe-derived metabolite trimethylamine N-oxide induces cardiac hypertrophy and fibrosis. *Lab. Investig. J. Tech. Methods Pathol.* **2019**, *99*, 346–357. [CrossRef] [PubMed]
72. Sun, X.; Jiao, X.; Ma, Y.; Liu, Y.; Zhang, L.; He, Y.; Chen, Y. Trimethylamine N-oxide induces inflammation and endothelial dysfunction in human umbilical vein endothelial cells via activating ROS-TXNIP-NLRP3 inflammasome. *Biochem. Biophys. Res. Commun.* **2016**, *481*, 63–70. [CrossRef] [PubMed]
73. Zhu, W.; Gregory, J.C.; Org, E.; Buffa, J.A.; Gupta, N.; Wang, Z.; Li, L.; Fu, X.; Wu, Y.; Mehrabian, M.; et al. Gut Microbial Metabolite TMAO Enhances Platelet Hyperreactivity and Thrombosis Risk. *Cell* **2016**, *165*, 111–124. [CrossRef]
74. Wang, G.; Kong, B.; Shuai, W.; Fu, H.; Jiang, X.; Huang, H. 3,3-Dimethyl-1-butanol attenuates cardiac remodeling in pressure-overload-induced heart failure mice. *J. Nutr. Biochem.* **2020**, *78*, 108341. [CrossRef]
75. Seldin, M.M.; Meng, Y.; Qi, H.; Zhu, W.; Wang, Z.; Hazen, S.L.; Lusis, A.J.; Shih, D.M. Trimethylamine N-Oxide Promotes Vascular Inflammation Through Signaling of Mitogen-Activated Protein Kinase and Nuclear Factor-κB. *J. Am. Heart Assoc.* **2016**, *5*, e002767. [CrossRef]

76. Savi, M.; Bocchi, L.; Bresciani, L.; Falco, A.; Quaini, F.; Mena, P.; Brighenti, F.; Crozier, A.; Stilli, D.; Del Rio, D. Trimethylamine-N-Oxide (TMAO)-Induced Impairment of Cardiomyocyte Function and the Protective Role of Urolithin B-Glucuronide. *Molecules* **2018**, *23*, 549. [CrossRef]
77. Chen, M.I.; Zhu, X.H.; Ran, L.; Lang, H.D.; Yi, L.; Mi, M.T. Trimethylamine-N-Oxide Induces Vascular Inflammation by Activating the NLRP3 Inflammasome Through the SIRT3-SOD2-mtROS Signaling Pathway. *J. Am. Heart Assoc.* **2017**, *6*, e006347. [CrossRef] [PubMed]
78. Suzuki, T.; Heaney, L.M.; Bhandari, S.S.; Jones, D.J.; Ng, L.L. Trimethylamine N-oxide and prognosis in acute heart failure. *Heart* **2016**, *102*, 841–848. [CrossRef] [PubMed]
79. Janeiro, M.H.; Ramírez, M.J.; Milagro, F.I.; Martínez, J.A.; Solas, M. Implication of Trimethylamine N-Oxide (TMAO) in Disease: Potential Biomarker or New Therapeutic Target. *Nutrients* **2018**, *10*, 1398. [CrossRef] [PubMed]
80. Tang, W.H.; Wang, Z.; Fan, Y.; Levison, B.; Hazen, J.E.; Donahue, L.M.; Wu, Y.; Hazen, S.L. Prognostic value of elevated levels of intestinal microbe-generated metabolite trimethylamine-N-oxide in patients with heart failure: Refining the gut hypothesis. *J. Am. Coll Cardiol.* **2014**, *64*, 1908–1914. [CrossRef]
81. Tang, W.H.W.; Wang, Z.; Shrestha, K.; Borowski, A.G.; Wu, Y.; Troughton, R.W.; Klein, A.L.; Hazen, S.L. Intestinal microbiota-dependent phosphatidylcholine metabolites, diastolic dysfunction, and adverse clinical outcomes in chronic systolic heart failure. *J. Card. Fail.* **2015**, *21*, 91–96. [CrossRef] [PubMed]

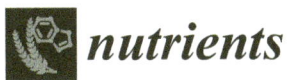

Review

Intake of Fish and Marine n-3 Polyunsaturated Fatty Acids and Risk of Cardiovascular Disease Mortality: A Meta-Analysis of Prospective Cohort Studies

Lan Jiang, Jinyu Wang, Ke Xiong, Lei Xu, Bo Zhang and Aiguo Ma *

Institute of Nutrition and Health, School of Public Health, Qingdao University, Qingdao 266071, China; jiangl59@163.com (L.J.); wangjinyu@qdu.edu.cn (J.W.); kexiong@qdu.edu.cn (K.X.); xulei951121@163.com (L.X.); zhangzhang19940516@163.com (B.Z.)
* Correspondence: magfood@qdu.edu.cn

Abstract: Previous epidemiological studies have investigated the association of fish and marine n-3 polyunsaturated fatty acids (n-3 PUFA) consumption with cardiovascular disease (CVD) mortality risk. However, the results were inconsistent. The purpose of this meta-analysis is to quantitatively evaluate the association between marine n-3 PUFA, fish and CVD mortality risk with prospective cohort studies. A systematic search was performed on PubMed, Web of Science, Embase and MEDLINE databases from the establishment of the database to May 2021. A total of 25 cohort studies were included with 2,027,512 participants and 103,734 CVD deaths. The results indicated that the fish consumption was inversely associated with the CVD mortality risk [relevant risk (RR) = 0.91; 95% confidence intervals (CI) 0.85−0.98]. The higher marine n-3 PUFA intake was associated with the reduced risk of CVD mortality (RR = 0.87; 95% CI: 0.85–0.89). Dose-response analysis suggested that the risk of CVD mortality was decreased by 4% with an increase of 20 g of fish intake (RR = 0.96; 95% CI: 0.94–0.99) or 80 milligrams of marine n-3 PUFA intake (RR = 0.96; 95% CI: 0.94–0.98) per day. The current work provides evidence that the intake of fish and marine n-3 PUFA are inversely associated with the risk of CVD mortality.

Keywords: fish; n-3 polyunsaturated fatty acid; cardiovascular disease mortality; meta-analysis; prospective cohort studies

Citation: Jiang, L.; Wang, J.; Xiong, K.; Xu, L.; Zhang, B.; Ma, A. Intake of Fish and Marine n-3 Polyunsaturated Fatty Acids and Risk of Cardiovascular Disease Mortality: A Meta-Analysis of Prospective Cohort Studies. *Nutrients* 2021, *13*, 2342. https://doi.org/10.3390/nu13072342

Academic Editor: Hayato Tada

Received: 21 May 2021
Accepted: 4 July 2021
Published: 9 July 2021

Publisher's Note: MDPI stays neutral with regard to jurisdictional claims in published maps and institutional affiliations.

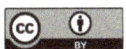

Copyright: © 2021 by the authors. Licensee MDPI, Basel, Switzerland. This article is an open access article distributed under the terms and conditions of the Creative Commons Attribution (CC BY) license (https://creativecommons.org/licenses/by/4.0/).

1. Introduction

Cardiovascular diseases (CVD) are a group of disorders of the heart and blood vessels, including coronary heart disease, cerebrovascular disease, rheumatic heart disease and other conditions. The global CVD mortality increased 12.5% from 2005 to 2015. 17.9 million people died of CVD in 2015 [1]. In addition to drug treatment, the potential role of dietary components has received increased attention. Previous studies have shown the effectiveness of healthy dietary patterns and components for the prevention of CVD and other diseases [2–4]. Fish is rich in various nutrients (e.g., protein, vitamin D and polyunsaturated fatty acids) and may have a beneficial role in preventing CVD events [5,6].

Marine n-3 polyunsaturated fatty acids (n-3 PUFA)—including eicosapentaenoic acid (EPA), docosahexaenoic acid (DHA) and docosapentaenoic acid (DPA)—mainly exist in fatty fish. A high consumption of n-3 PUFA from fatty fish led to an increase in high-density lipoprotein and a decrease in inflammation factors [7,8]. Besides, n-3 PUFA may improve heart rate and blood pressure through improving left ventricular diastolic filling or augmenting vagal tone [9].

Previous epidemiological studies have investigated the association of fish consumption with CVD mortality risk [10,11]. A recent meta-analysis of prospective observational studies revealed a negative association between fish intake and CVD mortality risk [12]. In recent years, another 11 prospective cohort studies investigated the association between fish intake and CVD mortality risk, but the findings were inconsistent [13–16]. The EPIC-Netherlands cohort study suggested that fish was not associated with the risk of CVD mortality [17]. In contrast, the NIH-AARP Diet and Health Study found that fish had a protective effect on CVD mortality risk [18]. To our knowledge, there has been no meta-analysis of prospective observational studies for investigating the association of marine n-3 PUFA consumption with CVD mortality risk. Therefore, we conducted this meta-analysis to comprehensively investigate the associations between fish, marine n-3 PUFA intake and CVD mortality risk. Furthermore, dose-response analyses were conducted to quantify the associations.

2. Materials and Methods

2.1. Data Sources and Search Strategy

Systematic search was performed on PubMed, Web of Science, Embase and MEDLINE from the establishment to May 2021. The search was limited to English literature, and the search keywords were "fish", "seafood", "fish products", "fish oil", "EPA", "eicosapentaenoic acid", "DHA", "docosahexaenoic acid", "DPA", "docosapentaenoic acid", "n-3 polyunsaturated fatty acid", "ω-3 polyunsaturated fatty acid", "n-3 PUFA", "ω-3 PUFA", "cardiovascular diseases", "CVD", "cardiovascular", "cohort", "follow-up", "prospective" and "longitudinal".

2.2. Study Selection

Two project members (L.J. and B.Z.) independently screened all titles and abstracts of the retrieved studies. Disagreements regarding the inclusion of the studies and the interpretation of the data were resolved by discussion among investigators. The studies were included in this meta-analysis if they met the following criteria: (1) study design: prospective cohort studies; (2) exposure: fish and marine n-3 PUFA; (3) source of n-3 PUFA: marine-derived n-3 PUFA (DHA, DPA, and EPA); and (4) outcomes: total CVD mortality which was reported as multivariate-adjusted relative risk (RR) and 95% confidence intervals (CI). The studies were excluded with the following criteria: (1) irrelevant; (2) not human studies; (3) not cohort studies; (4) not English studies.

2.3. Data Extraction

The following information was extracted from each eligible study: first author's surname; the year of publication; country; age; follow-up duration; the number of CVD deaths, sample size; gender; exposure levels; multivariate-adjusted RR with 95% CI for the highest versus the lowest category of fish or marine n-3 PUFA intake; adjusted covariates. Consumption of fish and marine n-3 PUFA was collected with adjusted RR (95% CI) to conduct dose-response analyses. Newcastle–Ottawa Quality Assessment Scale (NOS) was adopted to evaluate the quality of each included study [19]. The NOS score ranges from 0 (bad) to 9 (good).

The quality evaluation was performed independently by two project members (L.J. and B.Z.). The NOS quality score system assessed 3 items: population selection, comparability of the groups and outcome assessment. Any discrepancies in grading the quality were addressed by group discussion.

2.4. Statistical Analyses

All statistical analyses were performed using Stata (Version 15.1). RRs with 95% CI for all the exposure categories were extracted for the analysis. The main effect was RRs with 95% CI. A two-tailed $p < 0.05$ was considered as statistically significant. The summary estimation was conducted through the comparison of the highest and the lowest category. Heterogeneity was assessed using the I^2 statistic. In the case of heterogeneity for $I^2 > 50\%$, a random-effect model was adopted to pool the results. Otherwise, a fixed effect model was chosen.

Sensitivity analysis was implemented by deleting one study at a time. Subgroup analyses and meta-regression were performed to identify the possible sources of heterogeneity. In the subgroup analyses, the included studies were stratified by location (Asia, Europe plus America, Oceania and Five Continents), follow-up duration (<9 and ≥9 years), etc. In meta-regression, gender, country, dropout rate, follow-up duration, CVD history, adjustment for diabetes and adjustment for smoking were used as the covariates. Potential publication bias was accessed using funnel plots and Egger's test ($p < 0.1$ was considered statistically significant).

Non-linear dose-response analyses were performed to evaluate the relationship between fish, marine n-3 PUFA intake and CVD mortality risk [20]. Potential non-linear correlation was accessed by modeling the consumption level using restricted cubic splines. The distribution of four fixed knots were 5%, 35%, 65% and 95% [21]. Owing to the discrepancy of fish and marine n-3 PUFA intake categories, we selected studies with clear doses to perform dose-response analyses. Among each study, we used the median or mean consumption of fish and marine n-3 PUFA from each category. For open-ended categories, we set the lower boundary to zero in lowest category and the width of the category to be the same as the adjacent interval in the highest one [12,22].

3. Results

3.1. Literature Search and Study Characteristics

The process of literature search is presented in Figure 1. A total of 11,120 articles were identified. After screening the title and abstract, forty-five studies were selected for full-text evaluation. By full-text examination, twenty-five articles were eventually included for data synthesis with 2,027,512 participants and 103,734 CVD deaths [11,13–18,23–40].

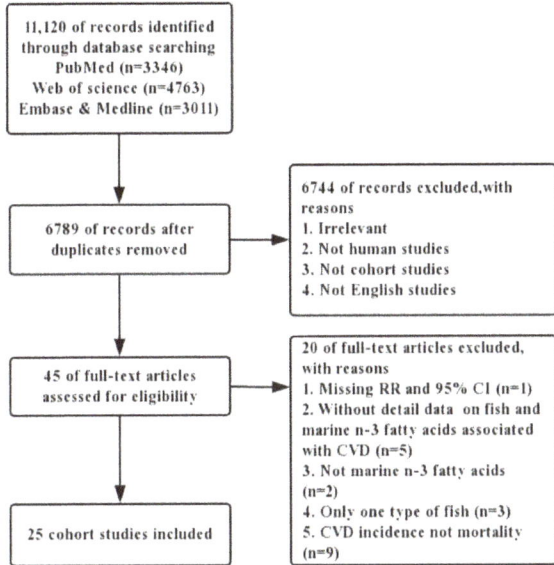

Figure 1. The flowchart for detailed steps of literature search.

The characteristics of the included studies are shown in Tables 1 and 2. Among these articles, sixteen were from Europe and America, seven from Asia, one from Oceania and one from five continents. The range of the age was 18–84 years old. The population in the study included males and females. Besides, follow-up duration ranged from 5–30 years and the NOS quality score ranged from 6–9 points (Tables S1 and S2).

Table 1. General characteristics of the studies included in meta-analysis of fish intake and risk of CVD mortality.

Author Name, Year, Country	Age Range/Mean Age (y)	Follow-Up Duration	Number of Cases/Size	Gender	Quantile	Adjusted RR (95% CI)	Quality Score	Adjustments
Mohan 2021, Asia, Africa, America, Europe and Oceania [40]	54.1	7.5	6502/191,454	M/F	4	0.85 (0.77–0.94)	6	Age, sex, study center, BMI, educational level, smoking status, alcohol intake, physical activity, urban or rural location, history of diabetes, cancer, use of statin or antihypertension medications, and intake of fruit, vegetables, red meat, poultry, dairy, and total energy
Kobayashi 2019, Japan [13]	45–74	14.9	2942/79,904	M/F	5	1.14 (0.99–1.32)	9	Age, area, BMI, alcohol intake total energy intake, coffee intake, green tea intake, smoking status, physical activity, occupation type, solitude and other food group
Kondo 2019, Japan [15]	30–79	29	1070/9115	M/F	3	0.72 (0.57–0.91)	8	Age, sex, smoking status, drinking status, and total energy intake
Van den brandt 2019, The Netherlands [16]	55–69	10	2985/120,852	M/F	4	1.45 (1.20–1.74)	9	Age at baseline, sex, cigarette smoking status, number of cigarettes smoked per day, years of smoking, diabetes, body height, non-occupational physical activity, highest level of education, intake of alcohol, vegetables and fruit, use of nutritional supplements and, in women, postmenopausal HRT
Deng 2018, USA [14]	≥18	18	326/1136	M/F	3	0.69 (0.50–0.96)	7	Age, sex, race/ethnicity, family income, the type of residential area, cigarette smoking, alcohol drinking, and the history of cardiovascular disease assessed at the baseline survey, and the years of using insulin as the indicator of diabetes severity
Hengeveld 2018, The Netherlands [17]	20–70	18	540/34,033	M/F	3	0.94 (0.80–1.10)	9	Age, sex, physical activity, smoking status, education level, BMI, alcohol intake, total energy intake, intakes of saturated fatty acids, trans fatty acids, fruit, vegetables, and dietary fiber
Zhang 2018, USA [18]	50–71	16	14824/240,729	M/F	5	0.9 (0.86–0.94)	8	Age, BMI, race, education, marital status, smoking, alcohol, intake of total energy, red meat, saturated fat, vegetables and fruits, multi-vitamin use, aspirin use, history of diabetes, history of hypertension, history of high cholesterol level
Bellavia 2017, Sweden [23]	45–83	17	5039/72,522	M/F	5	0.95 (0.94–0.95)	9	BMI, total physical activity, smoking status and pack-years of smoking, alcohol consumption, educational level (primary school, secondary school or university), total energy intake, fruit consumption, vegetable consumption, processed red meat consumption and non-processed red meat consumption
Nahab 2016, USA [24]	≥40	5.1	582/16,479	M/F	4	1.46 (0.87–2.45)	7	Age, race, region, sex, income, education, exercise, smoking status, Mediterranean diet score, regular aspirin use, total energy intake (kcald^{-1}), current use of hypertensive medication, diabetes status, systolic blood pressure, BMI and dyslipidaemia

Table 1. Cont.

Author Name, Year, Country	Age Range/Mean Age (y)	Follow-Up Duration	Number of Cases/Size	Gender	Quantile	Adjusted RR (95% CI)	Quality Score	Adjustments
Owen 2016, Australia [25]	≥25	9.7	277/11,247	M/F	4	0.66 (0.46–0.96)	7	Age, previous CVD, education, exercise, diabetes, total dietary energy and smoking
Eguchi 2014, Japan [26]	40–79	19.3	2412/42,946	M/F	2	0.89 (0.82–0.97)	8	Age, body mass index, history of hypertension, history of diabetes, education level, regular employment, perceived mental stress, and 7 health behaviors
Takata 2013, China [27]	40–74	8.7	1789/134,296	M/F	5	0.86 (0.70–1.05)	6	Age at baseline, total energy intake, income, occupation, education, comorbidity index, physical activity level, red meat intake, poultry intake, total vegetable intake, total fruit intake, smoking history, and alcohol consumption
Tomasallo 2010, USA [28]	45.8	12	44/1367	M/F	3	0.45 (0.21–0.99)	7	Age, sex, body mass index, and income at study baseline
Yamagishi 2008, Japan [29]	40–79	12.7	2045/57,972	M/F	5	0.82 (0.71–0.95)	7	Age, gender, history of hypertension and diabetes mellitus, smoking status, alcohol consumption, body mass index, mental stress, walking, sports, education levels, total energy, and dietary intakes of cholesterol, saturated and n-6 polyunsaturated fatty acids, vegetables, and fruit
Folsom 2004, USA [30]	55–69	14	1589/41,836	F	5	0.95 (0.78–1.15)	7	Age, energy intake, educational level, physical activity level, alcohol consumption, smoking status, pack-years of cigarette smoking, age at first livebirth, estrogen use, vitamin use, body mass index, waist/hip ratio, diabetes, hypertension, intake of whole grains, fruit and vegetables, red meat, cholesterol, and saturated fat
Gillum 2000, USA [31]	25–74	18.8	–/8825	M/F	4	1.01 (0.81–1.25)	9	Age, smoking, history of diabetes, education, high school graduate, systolic blood pressure, serum cholesterol concentration, body mass index, alcohol intake, and physical activity
Albert 1998 [32]	40–84	11	548/20,551	M	5	0.81 (0.49–1.33)	8	Age, aspirin and beta carotene treatment assignment, evidence of cardiovascular disease, prior to 12-month questionnaire, body mass index, smoking status, history of diabetes, history of hypertension, history of hypercholesterolemia, alcohol consumption, vigorous exercise, and vitamin E, vitamin C, and multivitamin use
Daviglus 1997 [33]	40–55	30	573/2107	M	4	0.74 (0.52–1.06)	8	Age, education, religion, systolic pressure, serum cholesterol, number of cigarettes smoked per day, body-mass index, presence or absence of diabetes, presence or absence of electrocardiographic abnormalities, daily intake of energy, cholesterol, saturated, monounsaturated, and polyunsaturated fatty acids, total protein, carbohydrate, alcohol, iron, thiamine, riboflavin, niacin, vitamin C, beta carotene, and retinol

CVD, cardiovascular disease; BMI, body mass index; HRT, hormone replacement therapy.

Table 2. General characteristics of the studies included in meta-analysis of marine n-3 PUFA intake and risk of CVD mortality.

Author Name, Year, Country	Age Range/Mean Age (y)	Follow-Up Duration	Number of Cases/Size	Gender	Quantile	Adjusted RR (95% CI)	Quality Score	Adjustments
Donat-Varga 2020, Sweden [34]	Men: 65.5 Women: 62.5	15.5	6338/69,497	M/F	5	0.79 (0.66–0.95)	8	Age, gender, education level, waist circumference, hypertension, hypercholesterolemia, weight loss > 5kg within 1 year, leisure-time inactivity and daily walking/cycling, family history of myocardial infarction before the age of 60 years, smoking status, use of aspirin, energy intake, Mediterranean diet, parity, use of hormone replacement therapy and dietary methylmercury exposure, dietary PCB exposure
Zhuang 2019, USA [35]	50–71	16	38,747/521,120	M/F	5	0.9 (0.87–0.94)	8	Age, gender, BMI, race, education, marital status, household income, smoking, alcohol drinking, physical activity, multi-vitamin use, aspirin use, history of hypertension, history of hypercholesterolemia, perceived health condition, history of heart disease, stroke, diabetes, and cancer at baseline, hormones use for women, intake of total energy, percentages of energy intake from protein, and remaining fatty acids where appropriate (saturated, α-linolenic, marine omega-3, linoleic, arachidonic, monounsaturated and trans fatty acids)
Zhang 2018, USA [18]	50–71	16	22,365/421,309	M/F	5	0.84 (0.80–0.88)	8	Age, BMI, race, education, marital status, smoking, alcohol, intake of total energy, red meat, saturated fat, vegetables and fruits, physical activity, multi-vitamin use, aspirin use, history of diabetes, history of hypertension, history of high cholesterol level and hormones use, intake of α-linolenic acid, omega-6 PUFAs, monounsaturated fatty acids and trans-fatty acid
Rhee 2016, USA [11]	≥45	22	501/39,876	F	5	1.15 (0.87–1.51)	9	Age, BMI, smoking, alcohol intake, physical activity, randomized treatment, oral contraceptive use, use of hormones as defined under HRT, multivitamin use, family history of MI, baseline history of hypertension, high cholesterol, and diabetes, intakes of dietary fiber, fruits and vegetables, trans fat, ratio of polyunsaturated to saturated fat, and sodium
Owen 2016, Australia [25]	≥25	9.7	277/11,247	M/F	5	1.00 (0.62–1.60)	7	Age, sex, previous CVD, education, exercise, diabetes, total dietary energy and smoking
Miyagawa 2014, Japan [36]	≥30	24	879/9190	M/F	4	0.80 (0.66–0.96)	7	Age, sex, smoking status, drinking status, systolic blood pressure, blood glucose, serum total cholesterol, body mass index, antihypertensive medication status, residential area, dietary intakes of saturated fatty acids, total n-6 PUFA, vegetable protein, total dietary fiber and sodium

Table 2. Cont.

Author Name, Year, Country	Age Range/Mean Age (y)	Follow-Up Duration	Number of Cases/Size	Gender	Quantile	Adjusted RR (95% CI)	Quality Score	Adjustments
Bell 2014, USA [37]	50–76	5	769/70,495	M/F	4	0.87 (0.68–1.10)	6	Age, sex, race/ethnicity, marital status, education, body mass index, physical activity, smoking, alcohol intake, total energy intake, vegetables intake, dietary intake of arachidonic acid, aspirin use, use of non-aspirin nonsteroidal anti-inflammatory drugs, self-rated health, sigmoidoscopy, mammogram, prostate-specific antigen test, current use of cholesterol-lowering medication, history of cardiovascular disease, family history of heart attack, current use of blood pressure medication, percentage of calories derived from trans-fat, percentage of calories derived from saturated fat, years of estrogen therapy, and years of estrogen + progestin therapy etc.
Koh 2013, Singapore [38]	45–74	14.8	4780/60,298	M/F	4	0.86 (0.77–0.96)	8	Age, sex, dialect, year of interview, educational level, body mass index, physical activity, smoking status, alcohol use, baseline history of self-reported diabetes, hypertension, coronary heart disease, stroke, and total energy, adjusted for intakes of protein, dietary fiber, monounsaturated fat, saturated fat, omega-6 fatty acids, and alternate omega-3 fatty acids
Takata 2013, China [27]	40–74	8.7	1789/134,296	M/F	5	0.74 (0.62–0.88)	6	Age, total energy intake, income, occupation, education, comorbidity index, physical activity level, red meat intake, poultry intake, total vegetable intake, total fruit intake, smoking history, and alcohol consumption (among men only)
Kamphuis 2006, The Netherlands [39]	70–79	10	92/332	M	3	0.88 (0.51–1.5)	8	Age, years of education, BMI, smoking, alcohol consumption, systolic blood pressure, total and HDL–cholesterol concentrations, physical activity, living alone, and energy intake

n-3 PUFA, n-3 polyunsaturated fatty acid; CVD, cardiovascular disease; PCB, polychlorinated biphenyl; BMI, body mass index; HRT, hormone replacement therapy; MI, myocardial infarction.

3.2. Fish Consumption and Cardiovascular Disease Mortality Risk

Eighteen studies, involving 1,267,951 participants and 51,628 CVD deaths, investigated the association between the fish intake and the CVD mortality risk [13–18,23–33,40]. The pooled RR (95% CI) was 0.91 (0.85–0.98) for the highest versus the lowest fish consumption category (I^2 = 70.0%) (Figure 2). Sensitivity analysis did not change the protective effects of fish on CVD mortality (Figure S1). Subgroup analysis suggested that there was a significant negative association between the fish intake and the CVD mortality risk among the subgroups with nine years or more follow-up duration (Table 3). No publication bias was found (Egger's test: p = 0.919; funnel plot: Figure S2).

Figure 3a showed the linear and non-linear dose-response analyses between the fish intake and the CVD mortality risk. Ten prospective cohort studies met the requirements for dose-response analysis [13,15–18,23,27,29,33,40], and the curvilinear correlation presented a downward trend for the adjusted RR of CVD deaths with the increase of fish consumption from zero to 40 g/d ($p_{\text{non-linearity}}$ < 0.001). The adjusted RR reached a steady value when fish consumption increased beyond 40 g/d. In the linear dose-response analysis, the summary RR (95% CI) for a 20 g/d increment was 0.96 (0.94–0.99) for CVD mortality risk (p_{trend} = 0.002).

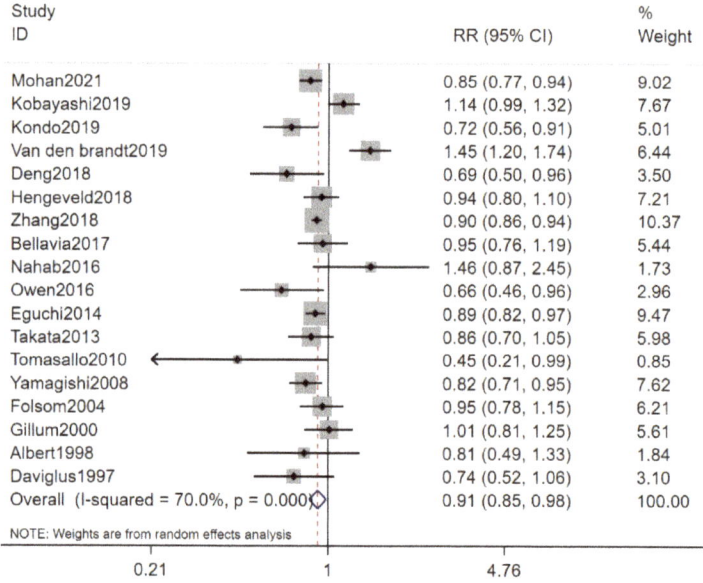

Figure 2. Forest plot of the highest versus lowest fish intake category and CVD mortality risk. Plot demonstrates decreased risk of CVD mortality risk with fish intake by the random-effects model (RR = 0.91; 95% CI, 0.85–0.98). CVD, cardiovascular disease; RR, relevant risk; CI, confidence intervals.

3.3. Marine n-3 PUFA and Cardiovascular Disease Mortality Risk

Ten eligible studies with 1,337,660 participants and 76,537 CVD deaths explored the association of marine n-3 PUFA intake with CVD mortality risk [11,18,25,27,34–39]. The pooled RR (95% CI) for the highest versus the lowest marine n-3 PUFA consumption category was 0.87 (0.85–0.89), with a low heterogeneity (I^2 = 37.8%) (Figure 4). Sensitivity analysis suggested a great impact on one article with high quality (Figure S3) [35]. The negative association between marine n-3 PUFA and the risk of CVD mortality was altered from 0.87 (0.85–0.89) to 0.84 (0.81–0.87) by deleting this study. Subgroup analyses displayed a significant negative association among the Americas, and Asian and European countries compared with Oceania countries (Table 3). No publication bias was found (Egger's test: $p = 0.722$; funnel plot: Figure S4). Figure 3b showed the linear and non-linear dose-response analysis between marine n-3 PUFA intake and CVD mortality risk. Eight prospective cohort studies met the requirements of dose-response analysis [18,25,27,34,36–39], and the curvilinear correlation presented a downward trend of CVD deaths with the increase of n-3 PUFA intake ($p_{\text{non-linearity}} < 0.001$). Linear dose-response analysis suggested that an increase of 80 milligrams of n-3 PUFA per day was associated with a 4% lower risk of CVD mortality (95% CI: 0.94–0.98; $p_{\text{trend}} < 0.001$).

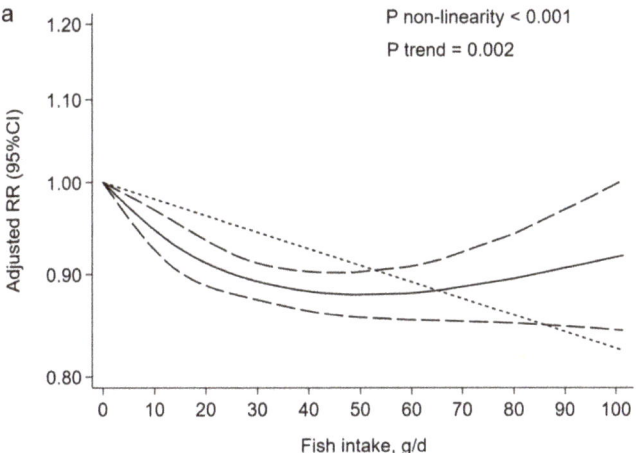

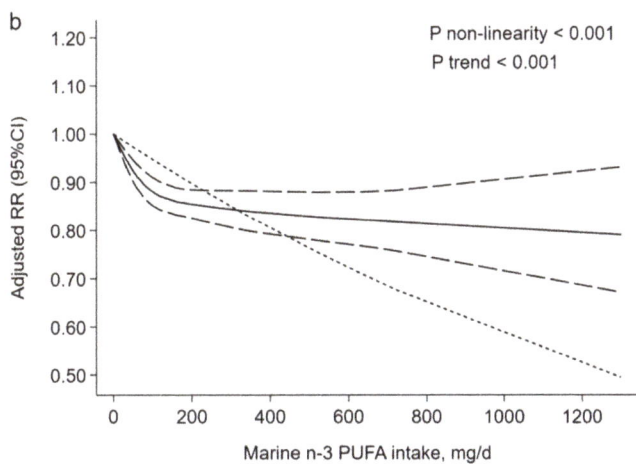

Figure 3. Dose-response association: (**a**) fish and CVD mortality ($n = 10$, $p_{\text{non-linearity}} < 0.001$; $p_{\text{trend}} = 0.002$); the risk of CVD mortality was decreased by 4% with an increase of 20 g of fish intake (RR = 0.96; 95% CI: 0.94–0.99) per day. (**b**) marine n-3 PUFA and CVD mortality ($n = 8$, $p_{\text{non-linearity}} < 0.001$; $p_{\text{trend}} < 0.001$); the risk of CVD mortality was decreased by 4% with an increase of 80 milligrams of marine n-3 PUFA intake (RR = 0.96; 95% CI: 0.94–0.98) per day. CVD, cardiovascular disease; n-3 PUFA, n-3 polyunsaturated fatty acids; RR, relevant risk; CI, confidence intervals; g/d, grams per day; mg/d, milligrams per day.

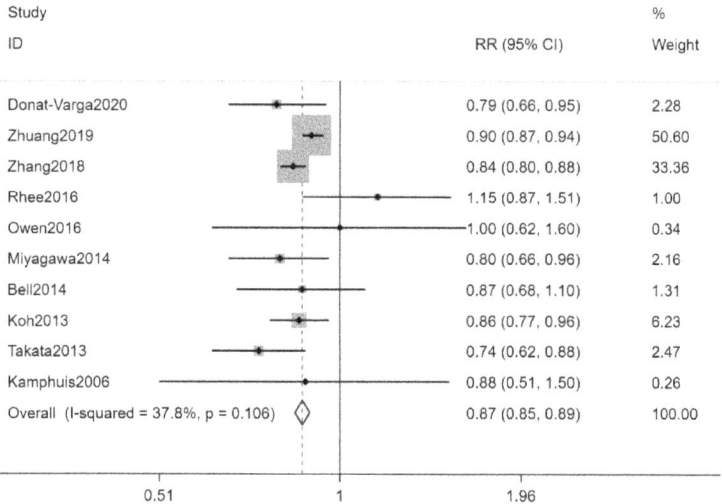

Figure 4. Forest plot of the highest versus lowest marine n-3 PUFA intake category and CVD mortality risk. Plot demonstrates decreased risk of CVD mortality risk with n-3 PUFA intake by the fixed-effects model (RR = 0.87; 95% CI, 0.85–0.89). CVD, cardiovascular disease; n-3 PUFA, n-3 polyunsaturated fatty acids; RR, relevant risk; CI, confidence intervals.

Table 3. Subgroup and meta-regression analyses for the association between fish, n-3 PUFA intake and CVD mortality.

Comparison		N [†]	Pooled RRs (95% CI)	Heterogeneity (I^2), p^a Value	p^b Value	p^c Value
Fish Intake and CVD Mortality Risk		18	0.91 (0.85–0.98)	70.0%, 0.000	0.015	
Country	Asia	5	0.89 (0.78–1.01)	74.1%, 0.004	0.081	
	Europe and America	11	0.95 (0.84–1.08)	72.2%, 0.000	0.417	0.216
	Oceania	1	0.66 (0.46–0.95)	–	0.027	
	Asia, Africa, America, Europe and Oceania	1	0.85 (0.77, 0.94)	–	0.001	
Gender	Men	2	0.76 (0.57–1.02)	0.0%, 0.773	0.067	
	women	1	0.95 (0.78–1.15)	–	0.605	0.442
	Both	15	0.92 (0.85–1.00)	74.5%, 0.000	0.040	
Follow-up duration	<9 years	3	0.90 (0.76–1.07)	50.6%, 0.132	0.234	0.851
	≥9 years	15	0.91 (0.84–0.99)	72.7%, 0.000	0.035	
Dropout rate	<20%	11	0.93 (0.82–1.06)	76.7%, 0.000	0.284	0.557
	>20%	7	0.88 (0.82–0.94)	41.6%, 0.113	0.000	
Excluding history of CVD	Yes	11	0.97 (0.88–1.06)	77.0%, 0.000	0.492	0.905
	No	7	0.82 (0.75–0.91)	21.7%, 0.264	0.000	
Adjustment for diabetes	Yes	11	0.93 (0.85, 1.01)	72.9%, 0.000	0.094	
	No	4	0.84 (0.63, 1.12)	80.9%, 0.001	0.233	0.040
	Others *	3	0.89 (0.76, 1.04)	34.5%, 0.217	0.149	
Adjustment for smoking	Yes	16	0.92 (0.85, 1.00)	71.8%, 0.000	0.050	0.484
	No	2	0.71 (0.38, 1.33)	66.0%, 0.087	0.285	
Marine n-3 PUFA and CVD mortality risk		10	0.87 (0.85–0.89)	37.8%, 0.106	0.000	
Country	Asia	3	0.82 (0.75–0.89)	4.9%, 0.349	0.000	
	Europe and America	6	0.88 (0.85–0.90)	49.2%, 0.08	0.000	0.212
	Oceania	1	1.00 (0.62–1.61)	–	1.000	

Table 3. Cont.

Comparison		N [†]	Pooled RRs (95% CI)	Heterogeneity (I²), p [a] Value	p [b] Value	p [c] Value
Gender	Men	1	0.88 (0.51–1.51)	–	0.642	
	Women	1	1.15 (0.87–1.52)	–	0.320	0.182
	Both	8	0.87 (0.84–0.89)	33.3%, 0.162	0.000	
Follow-up duration	<9 years	2	0.78 (0.68–0.90)	12.1%, 0.286	0.001	0.192
	≥9 years	8	0.87 (0.85–0.90)	37.0%, 0.134	0.000	
Dropout rate	<20%	5	0.89 (0.86–0.92)	51.8%, 0.08	0.000	0.114
	>20%	5	0.84 (0.80–0.87)	0.0%, 0.877	0.000	
Excluding history of CVD	Yes	5	0.84 (0.81–0.88)	29.9%, 0.222	0.000	0.536
	No	5	0.89 (0.86–0.92)	23.4%, 0.266	0.000	
Adjustment for diabetes	Yes	6	0.88 (0.85, 0.90)	44.4%, 0.109	0.000	
	No	3	0.77 (0.68, 0.88)	0.0%, 0.745	0.000	0.060
	Others *	1	0.79 (0.66, 0.95)	–	0.0 11	

N [†] Number of included studies; p [a] for heterogeneity; p [b] for significance test; p [c] for meta-regression analysis. Others * All patients were diabetic or not diabetic. n-3 PUFA, n-3 polyunsaturated fatty acid; CVD, cardiovascular disease.

4. Discussion

To our knowledge, the current work is the first meta-analysis of prospective observational studies for associating marine n-3 PUFA intake and CVD mortality risk. This study showed a significant inverse association between fish, marine n-3 PUFA intake and CVD mortality risk. Nonlinear dose-response relationship found that an increase of 20 g of fish intake or 80 milligrams of marine n-3 PUFA intake per day was associated with a 4% reduction in risk of CVD mortality.

In accordance with the previous study, the fish consumption was inversely associated with the CVD mortality risk in the current meta-analysis [12]. Bechthold et al.'s study also suggested a negative association between fish consumption and the risk of CVD [41]. Several studies showed no association between the fish intake and the risk of CVD [42,43]. Differences in preparation and type of fish might explain the observed difference. The progress of frying deteriorates oils through oxidation and hydrogenation, leading to an increase of trans fatty acids [44]. Trans fatty acids can aggravate inflammation and endothelial dysfunction, increasing the risk of CVD mortality [45]. Fish high in salt during cooking can increase the risk of CVD through increasing production of reactive oxygen species and oxidative stress, which contribute to impaired vascular function [46,47]. Fish can be divided into lean, medium-fatty or fatty fish with less than 2 g, 2–8 g and more than 8 g fat per 100 g in its body tissue [48]. Fatty fish diets significantly decreased the serum concentrations of triacylglycerol, apolipoprotein B, apolipoprotein CII and apolipoprotein CIII, which were known CVD risk markers [49]. Fishes also contain vitamin D, proteins, minerals and taurine which may decrease markers of inflammation and improve vascular function by increasing adiponectin levels [50]. In the subgroup of adjustment for diabetes, fish intake was associated with a reduction in the rate of major CVD mortality that approached significance (RR = 0.93; 95% CI: 0.85–1.01). Previous study has showed that supplementation of fish can decrease the CVD mortality risk in a diabetic population [51], the possible reason being that diabetes is a significant risk factor for CVD mortality [52]. EPA and DHA derived from fish can activate the G protein–coupled receptor 120 to reverse insulin resistance [53]. n-3 PUFA supplementation can protect against CVD in patients with diabetes [54].

In most studies where fish exits as an exposure variable, the observed benefits could often be attributed to the presence of fatty acids [55,56]. The long chain n-3 PUFA—namely, EPA and DHA—are naturally presented not only in fatty fish, but also in lean fish [57,58]. n-3 PUFA supplementation can decrease the risk of CVD [59,60]. The plasma level of EPA and DHA in humans may increase after intake of fish to improve the composition of lipoprotein cholesterol as cardiovascular markers affecting the risk of CVD [61,62]. However, previous study showed that low-dose supplementation with EPA and DHA did not significantly reduce the rate of CVD events [63]. This possible reason may be related to presence or absence of a history of CVD. The patients in the trial were all myocardial infarction patients for 4 years before enrollment. 85% of the patients were receiving statins. Patients with CVD who are receiving good clinical treatment showed low risk of future cardiovascular events [64]. Therefore, we wanted to observe the effect of the long chain n-3 PUFA on CVD mortality through the long-term duration.

In this meta-analysis, we also found a negative association between the marine n-3 PUFA intake and the CVD mortality risk. In previous studies, the results were not consistent [65]. A randomized controlled trial (RCT) showed that n-3 PUFA supplementation (866 mg/d) for 3.5 years could reduce CVD mortality risk [66]. In contrast, the RCT with one-year n-3 PUFA supplementation (850 mg/d) suggested no association [67]. Although some randomized controlled trials (RCTs) had been published, the follow-up duration were short with most studies ranged from 1–5 years [66–68]. Hoverer, the cohort studies included in this meta-analysis have longer follow-up duration ranged from 5–29 years. CVD is a chronic disease with a long disease course. Longer follow-up duration was more in line with the nature of the CVD disease. The possible mechanisms were as follows. First, the plasma n-3 PUFA increased with the frequency and the amount of dietary n-3 PUFA intake [69,70]. A higher circulating n-3 PUFA may alter the cell membrane fluidity which modulates protein function and signaling. The dimerization and recruitment of toll-like receptor-4 may be disrupted to down-regulate the expression of nuclear factor-kappaB reducing the inflammatory responses, with the enrichment of n-3 PUFA [71]. Second, n-3 PUFA may inhibit oxidative stress through the nuclear factor E2-related factor 2/heme oxygenase-1 signaling pathway. 4-hydroxy-2E-hexenal, the product of n-3 PUFA peroxidation, will dissociate Nrf2 from Keap1 and react with the cysteine residues of Keap1 [72]. Then, Nrf2 can translocate into the nucleus and bind to antioxidant responsive element to increase the expression of HO-1 [73]. HO-1 is a representative antioxidant enzyme that can confer cytoprotection on a wide variety of cells against oxidative damage [72]. Third, n-3 PUFA may reduce the hepatic very low-density lipoprotein production rate to decrease the plasma triglyceride levels through affecting fatty acid desaturases, fatty acid elongases and peroxisomal β- gene expression and fatty acid beta-oxidation [74,75]. In addition, long-chain n-3 PUFA may play an important role in improving the endothelial function, lowering circulating markers of endothelial dysfunction, such as E-selectin, vascular cell adhesion molecule-1 and intercellular adhesion molecule-1 [76–78].

The dose–response analysis showed that the risk of CVD mortality decreased with the increase of fish consumption from zero to 40 g/d. The adjusted RR reached a steady value when fish consumption increased beyond 40 g/d. Therefore, we believe that 40 g/d is the ideal dose for preventing CVD mortality. This is basically consistent with the average fish intake of the population of Europe and America [23,30]. However, the average intake of people in Japan is higher than this level [13].

This study has several strengths. First, compared with the previous meta-analysis [12], this study included additional 11 studies to investigate the association between the fish consumption and the CVD mortality risk, which may have a higher statistical power. Second, this meta-analysis was first to investigate the association between marine n-3 PUFA intake and CVD mortality risk with prospective cohort studies. Third, most studies had a long follow-up duration (9–30 years). CVD is a chronic disease and longer follow-up duration can better explain the association between fish, marine n-3 PUFA and CVD mortality risk.

The limitations should be acknowledged. First, several deep-sea fishes may be contaminated, while only one article reported whether fishes had pollutants or not [28]. Second, it is hard to standardize the fish and marine n-3 PUFA consumption due to the details of measurement methods not being available. Thus, we chose RR (95% CI) of the highest versus lowest fish and marine n-3 PUFA intake category and CVD mortality risk.

5. Conclusions

This meta-analysis indicated that the fish and marine n-3 PUFA intake were inversely associated with reduced risk of CVD mortality. This finding has important public health implications in terms of the prevention of CVD mortality. Since the biomarkers of fish and n-3 PUFA within an individual are important for food absorption, further research needs to be performed in biomarkers.

Supplementary Materials: The following are available online at https://www.mdpi.com/article/10.3390/nu13072342/s1, Figure S1: Sensitivity analysis with respect to fish intake and CVD mortality risk. Figure S2: Funnel plot of the RR of 18 articles on fish intake and CVD mortality risk. Figure S3: Sensitivity analysis with respect to marine n-3 PUFA intake and CVD mortality risk. Figure S4: Funnel plot of the RR of 10 articles on marine n-3 PUFA intake and CVD mortality risk. Table S1: Quality assessment of studies investigating fish intake and CVD mortality risk. Table S2: Quality assessment of studies investigating marine n-3 PUFA intake and CVD mortality risk.

Author Contributions: L.J. and A.M. designed research; J.W., K.X., B.Z., L.X. and L.J. conducted research; L.J. analyzed data and wrote the paper. A.M. had primary responsibility for final content. All authors have read and agreed to the published version of the manuscript.

Funding: This research received no external funding.

Conflicts of Interest: The authors declare no conflict of interest.

References

1. Mortality, G.B.D.; Causes of Death, C. Global, regional, and national life expectancy, all-cause mortality, and cause-specific mortality for 249 causes of death, 1980-2015: A systematic analysis for the Global Burden of Disease Study 2015. *Lancet* **2016**, *388*, 1459–1544. [CrossRef]
2. Rosato, V.; Temple, N.J.; La Vecchia, C.; Castellan, G.; Tavani, A.; Guercio, V. Mediterranean diet and cardiovascular disease: A systematic review and meta-analysis of observational studies. *Eur. J. Nutr.* **2019**, *58*, 173–191. [CrossRef] [PubMed]
3. Wang, J.; Xiong, K.; Xu, L.; Zhang, C.; Zhao, S.; Liu, Y.; Ma, A. Dietary Intake of Vegetables and Cooking Oil Was Associated with Drug-Induced Liver Injury During Tuberculosis Treatment: A Preliminary Cohort Study. *Front. Nutr.* **2021**, *8*, 652311. [CrossRef] [PubMed]
4. Xiong, K.; Zhou, L.; Wang, J.; Ma, A.; Fang, D.; Xiong, L.; Sun, Q. Construction of food-grade pH-sensitive nanoparticles for delivering functional food ingredients. *Trends Food Sci. Technol.* **2020**, *96*, 102–113. [CrossRef]
5. Denissen, K.F.M.; Heil, S.G.; Eussen, S.; Heeskens, J.P.J.; Thijs, C.; Mommers, M.; Smits, L.J.M.; van Dongen, M.; Dagnelie, P.C. Intakes of Vitamin B-12 from Dairy Food, Meat, and Fish and Shellfish Are Independently and Positively Associated with Vitamin B-12 Biomarker Status in Pregnant Dutch Women. *J. Nutr.* **2019**, *149*, 131–138. [CrossRef]
6. Bergqvist, C.; Ezzedine, K. Vitamin D and the skin: What should a dermatologist know? *G. Ital. Dermatol. Venereol.* **2019**, *154*, 669–680. [CrossRef]
7. Hustad, K.S.; Rundblad, A.; Ottestad, I.; Christensen, J.J.; Holven, K.B.; Ulven, S.M. Comprehensive lipid and metabolite profiling in healthy adults with low and high consumption of fatty fish: A cross-sectional study. *Br. J. Nutr.* **2020**, 1–23. [CrossRef]
8. Asher, A.; Tintle, N.L.; Myers, M.; Lockshon, L.; Bacareza, H.; Harris, W.S. Blood omega-3 fatty acids and death from COVID-19: A pilot study. *Prostaglandins Leukot. Essent. Fat. Acids* **2021**, *166*, 102250. [CrossRef]
9. O'Keefe, J.H., Jr.; Abuissa, H.; Sastre, A.; Steinhaus, D.M.; Harris, W.S. Effects of omega-3 fatty acids on resting heart rate, heart rate recovery after exercise, and heart rate variability in men with healed myocardial infarctions and depressed ejection fractions. *Am. J. Cardiol.* **2006**, *97*, 1127–1130. [CrossRef]
10. Jayedi, A.; Shab-Bidar, S. Fish Consumption and the Risk of Chronic Disease: An Umbrella Review of Meta-Analyses of Prospective Cohort Studies. *Adv. Nutr.* **2020**. [CrossRef]
11. Rhee, J.J.; Kim, E.; Buring, J.E.; Kurth, T. Fish Consumption, Omega-3 Fatty Acids, and Risk of Cardiovascular Disease. *Am. J. Prev. Med.* **2017**, *52*, 10–19. [CrossRef] [PubMed]
12. Jayedi, A.; Shab-Bidar, S.; Eimeri, S.; Djafarian, K. Fish consumption and risk of all-cause and cardiovascular mortality: A dose-response meta-analysis of prospective observational studies. *Public Health Nutr.* **2018**, *21*, 1297–1306. [CrossRef] [PubMed]
13. Kobayashi, M.; Sasazuki, S.; Shimazu, T.; Sawada, N.; Yamaji, T.; Iwasaki, M.; Mizoue, T.; Tsugane, S. Association of dietary diversity with total mortality and major causes of mortality in the Japanese population: JPHC study. *Eur. J. Clin. Nutr.* **2020**, *74*, 54–66. [CrossRef] [PubMed]
14. Deng, A.; Pattanaik, S.; Bhattacharya, A.; Yin, J.; Ross, L.; Liu, C.; Zhang, J. Fish consumption is associated with a decreased risk of death among adults with diabetes: 18-year follow-up of a national cohort. *Nutr. Metab. Cardiovasc. Dis.* **2018**, *28*, 1012–1020. [CrossRef]

15. Kondo, K.; Miura, K.; Tanaka-Mizuno, S.; Kadota, A.; Arima, H.; Okuda, N.; Fujiyoshi, A.; Miyagawa, N.; Yoshita, K.; Okamura, T.; et al. Cardiovascular Risk Assessment Chart by Dietary Factors in Japan—NIPPON DATA80. *Circ. J.* **2019**, *83*, 1254–1260. [CrossRef]
16. van den Brandt, P.A. Red meat, processed meat, and other dietary protein sources and risk of overall and cause-specific mortality in The Netherlands Cohort Study. *Eur. J. Epidemiol.* **2019**, *34*, 351–369. [CrossRef]
17. Hengeveld, L.M.; Praagman, J.; Beulens, J.W.J.; Brouwer, I.A.; van der Schouw, Y.T.; Sluijs, I. Fish consumption and risk of stroke, coronary heart disease, and cardiovascular mortality in a Dutch population with low fish intake. *Eur. J. Clin. Nutr.* **2018**, *72*, 942–950. [CrossRef] [PubMed]
18. Zhang, Y.; Zhuang, P.; He, W.; Chen, J.N.; Wang, W.Q.; Freedman, N.D.; Abnet, C.C.; Wang, J.B.; Jiao, J.J. Association of fish and long-chain omega-3 fatty acids intakes with total and cause-specific mortality: Prospective analysis of 421 309 individuals. *J. Intern. Med.* **2018**, *284*, 399–417. [CrossRef]
19. Stang, A. Critical evaluation of the Newcastle-Ottawa scale for the assessment of the quality of nonrandomized studies in meta-analyses. *Eur. J. Epidemiol.* **2010**, *25*, 603–605. [CrossRef]
20. Orsini, N.; Bellocco, R.; Greenland, S. Generalized least squares for trend estimation of summarized dose–response data. *STATA J.* **2016**, *6*, 40–57. [CrossRef]
21. Greenland, S.; Longnecker, M.P. Methods for trend estimation from summarized dose-response data, with applications to meta-analysis. *Am. J. Epidemiol.* **1992**, *135*, 1301–1309. [CrossRef]
22. Wang, X.; Ouyang, Y.; Liu, J.; Zhu, M.; Zhao, G.; Bao, W.; Hu, F.B. Fruit and vegetable consumption and mortality from all causes, cardiovascular disease, and cancer: Systematic review and dose-response meta-analysis of prospective cohort studies. *BMJ* **2014**, *349*, g4490. [CrossRef]
23. Bellavia, A.; Larsson, S.C.; Wolk, A. Fish consumption and all-cause mortality in a cohort of Swedish men and women. *J. Intern. Med.* **2017**, *281*, 86–95. [CrossRef]
24. Nahab, F.; Pearson, K.; Frankel, M.R.; Ard, J.; Safford, M.M.; Kleindorfer, D.; Howard, V.J.; Judd, S. Dietary fried fish intake increases risk of CVD: The REasons for Geographic and Racial Differences in Stroke (REGARDS) study. *Public Health Nutr.* **2016**, *19*, 3327–3336. [CrossRef]
25. Owen, A.J.; Magliano, D.J.; O'Dea, K.; Barr, E.L.; Shaw, J.E. Polyunsaturated fatty acid intake and risk of cardiovascular mortality in a low fish-consuming population: A prospective cohort analysis. *Eur. J. Nutr.* **2016**, *55*, 1605–1613. [CrossRef]
26. Eguchi, E.; Iso, H.; Tanabe, N.; Yatsuya, H.; Tamakoshi, A. Is the association between healthy lifestyle behaviors and cardiovascular mortality modified by overweight status? The Japan Collaborative Cohort Study. *Prev. Med.* **2014**, *62*, 142–147. [CrossRef]
27. Takata, Y.; Zhang, X.; Li, H.; Gao, Y.T.; Yang, G.; Gao, J.; Cai, H.; Xiang, Y.B.; Zheng, W.; Shu, X.O. Fish intake and risks of total and cause-specific mortality in 2 population-based cohort studies of 134,296 men and women. *Am. J. Epidemiol.* **2013**, *178*, 46–57. [CrossRef]
28. Tomasallo, C.; Anderson, H.; Haughwout, M.; Imm, P.; Knobeloch, L. Mortality among frequent consumers of Great Lakes sport fish. *Environ. Res.* **2010**, *110*, 62–69. [CrossRef] [PubMed]
29. Yamagishi, K.; Iso, H.; Date, C.; Fukui, M.; Wakai, K.; Kikuchi, S.; Inaba, Y.; Tanabe, N.; Tamakoshi, A.; Grp, J.S. Fish, omega-3 polyunsaturated fatty acids, and mortality from cardiovascular diseases in a nationwide community-based cohort of Japanese men and women—The JACC (Japan Collaborative Cohort Study for Evaluation of Cancer Risk) study. *J. Am. Coll. Cardiol.* **2008**, *52*, 988–996. [CrossRef]
30. Folsom, A.R.; Demissie, Z. Fish intake, marine omega-3 fatty acids, and mortality in a cohort of postmenopausal women. *Am. J. Epidemiol.* **2004**, *160*, 1005–1010. [CrossRef]
31. Gillum, R.F.; Mussolino, M.; Madans, J.H. The relation between fish consumption, death from all causes, and incidence of coronary heart disease. the NHANES I Epidemiologic Follow-up Study. *J. Clin. Epidemiol.* **2000**, *53*, 237–244. [CrossRef]
32. Albert, C.M.; Hennekens, C.H.; O'Donnell, C.J.; Ajani, U.A.; Carey, V.J.; Willett, W.C.; Ruskin, J.N.; Manson, J.E. Fish consumption and risk of sudden cardiac death. *J. Am. Med. Assoc.* **1998**, *279*, 23–28. [CrossRef]
33. Daviglus, M.L.; Stamler, J.; Orencia, A.J.; Dyer, A.R.; Liu, K.; Greenland, P.; Walsh, M.K.; Morris, D.; Shekelle, R.B. Fish consumption and the 30-year risk of fatal myocardial infarction. *N. Engl. J. Med.* **1997**, *336*, 1046–1053. [CrossRef]
34. Donat-Vargas, C.; Bellavia, A.; Berglund, M.; Glynn, A.; Wolk, A.; Akesson, A. Cardiovascular and cancer mortality in relation to dietary polychlorinated biphenyls and marine polyunsaturated fatty acids: A nutritional-toxicological aspect of fish consumption. *J. Intern. Med.* **2020**, *287*, 197–209. [CrossRef]
35. Zhuang, P.; Zhang, Y.; He, W.; Chen, X.; Chen, J.; He, L.; Mao, L.; Wu, F.; Jiao, J. Dietary Fats in Relation to Total and Cause-Specific Mortality in a Prospective Cohort of 521 120 Individuals with 16 Years of Follow-Up. *Circ. Res.* **2019**, *124*, 757–768. [CrossRef]
36. Miyagawa, N.; Miura, K.; Okuda, N.; Kadowaki, T.; Takashima, N.; Nagasawa, S.Y.; Nakamura, Y.; Matsumura, Y.; Hozawa, A.; Fujiyoshi, A.; et al. Long-chain n-3 polyunsaturated fatty acids intake and cardiovascular disease mortality risk in Japanese: A 24-year follow-up of NIPPON DATA80. *Atherosclerosis* **2014**, *232*, 384–389. [CrossRef] [PubMed]
37. Bell, G.A.; Kantor, E.D.; Lampe, J.W.; Kristal, A.R.; Heckbert, S.R.; White, E. Intake of long-chain omega-3 fatty acids from diet and supplements in relation to mortality. *Am. J. Epidemiol.* **2014**, *179*, 710–720. [CrossRef] [PubMed]
38. Koh, A.S.; Pan, A.; Wang, R.; Odegaard, A.O.; Pereira, M.A.; Yuan, J.M.; Koh, W.P. The association between dietary omega-3 fatty acids and cardiovascular death: The Singapore Chinese Health Study. *Eur. J. Prev. Cardiol.* **2015**, *22*, 364–372. [CrossRef] [PubMed]

39. Kamphuis, M.H.; Geerlings, M.I.; Tijhuis, M.A.; Kalmijn, S.; Grobbee, D.E.; Kromhout, D. Depression and cardiovascular mortality: A role for n-3 fatty acids? *Am. J. Clin. Nutr.* **2006**, *84*, 1513–1517. [CrossRef]
40. Mohan, D.; Mente, A.; Dehghan, M.; Rangarajan, S.; O'Donnell, M.; Hu, W.; Dagenais, G.; Wielgosz, A.; Lear, S.; Wei, L.; et al. Associations of Fish Consumption with Risk of Cardiovascular Disease and Mortality Among Individuals with or Without Vascular Disease From 58 Countries. *JAMA Intern. Med.* **2021**, *181*, 631–649. [CrossRef]
41. Bechthold, A.; Boeing, H.; Schwedhelm, C.; Hoffmann, G.; Knuppel, S.; Iqbal, K.; De Henauw, S.; Michels, N.; Devleesschauwer, B.; Schlesinger, S.; et al. Food groups and risk of coronary heart disease, stroke and heart failure: A systematic review and dose-response meta-analysis of prospective studies. *Crit. Rev. Food Sci. Nutr.* **2019**, *59*, 1071–1090. [CrossRef]
42. Kuhn, T.; Teucher, B.; Kaaks, R.; Boeing, H.; Weikert, C.; Buijsse, B. Fish consumption and the risk of myocardial infarction and stroke in the German arm of the European Prospective Investigation into Cancer and Nutrition (EPIC-Germany). *Br. J. Nutr.* **2013**, *110*, 1118–1125. [CrossRef]
43. Myint, P.K.; Welch, A.A.; Bingham, S.A.; Luben, R.N.; Wareham, N.J.; Day, N.E.; Khaw, K.T. Habitual fish consumption and risk of incident stroke: The European Prospective Investigation into Cancer (EPIC)-Norfolk prospective population study. *Public Health Nutr.* **2006**, *9*, 882–888. [CrossRef]
44. Sun, Y.; Liu, B.; Snetselaar, L.G.; Robinson, J.G.; Wallace, R.B.; Peterson, L.L.; Bao, W. Association of fried food consumption with all cause, cardiovascular, and cancer mortality: Prospective cohort study. *BMJ* **2019**, *364*. [CrossRef] [PubMed]
45. Valenzuela, C.A.; Baker, E.J.; Miles, E.A.; Calder, P.C. Eighteencarbon trans fatty acids and inflammation in the context of atherosclerosis. *Prog. Lipid Res.* **2019**, *76*, 101009. [CrossRef]
46. He, F.J.; MacGregor, G.A. Role of salt intake in prevention of cardiovascular disease: Controversies and challenges. *Nat. Rev. Cardiol.* **2018**, *15*, 371–377. [CrossRef] [PubMed]
47. Lastra, G.; Dhuper, S.; Johnson, M.S.; Sowers, J.R. Salt, aldosterone, and insulin resistance: Impact on the cardiovascular system. *Nat. Rev. Cardiol.* **2010**, *7*, 577–584. [CrossRef]
48. VKM. Benefit-Risk Assessment of Fish and Fish Products in the Norwegian Diet—An Update. Scientific Opinion of the Scientific Steering Committee. VKM Report 15. Oslo, Norway, 2014; 293p, ISBN 978-82-8259-159-1. Available online: www.vkm.no (accessed on 25 April 2021).
49. Zhang, J.; Wang, C.; Li, L.; Man, Q.; Meng, L.; Song, P.; Froyland, L.; Du, Z.Y. Dietary inclusion of salmon, herring and pompano as oily fish reduces CVD risk markers in dyslipidaemic middle-aged and elderly Chinese women. *Br. J. Nutr.* **2012**, *108*, 1455–1465. [CrossRef]
50. Torris, C.; Smastuen, M.C.; Molin, M. Nutrients in Fish and Possible Associations with Cardiovascular Disease Risk Factors in Metabolic Syndrome. *Nutrients* **2018**, *10*, 952. [CrossRef]
51. Hu, F.B.; Cho, E.; Rexrode, K.M.; Albert, C.M.; Manson, J.E. Fish and long-chain omega-3 fatty acid intake and risk of coronary heart disease and total mortality in diabetic women. *Circulation* **2003**, *107*, 1852–1857. [CrossRef]
52. Wang, H.; Shara, N.M.; Lee, E.T.; Devereux, R.; Calhoun, D.; de Simone, G.; Umans, J.G.; Howard, B.V. Hemoglobin A1c, fasting glucose, and cardiovascular risk in a population with high prevalence of diabetes: The strong heart study. *Diabetes Care* **2011**, *34*, 1952–1958. [CrossRef]
53. Oh, D.Y.; Talukdar, S.; Bae, E.J.; Imamura, T.; Morinaga, H.; Fan, W.; Li, P.; Lu, W.J.; Watkins, S.M.; Olefsky, J.M. GPR120 is an omega-3 fatty acid receptor mediating potent anti-inflammatory and insulin-sensitizing effects. *Cell* **2010**, *142*, 687–698. [CrossRef]
54. Kromhout, D.; Geleijnse, J.M.; de Goede, J.; Oude Griep, L.M.; Mulder, B.J.; de Boer, M.J.; Deckers, J.W.; Boersma, E.; Zock, P.L.; Giltay, E.J. n-3 fatty acids, ventricular arrhythmia-related events, and fatal myocardial infarction in postmyocardial infarction patients with diabetes. *Diabetes Care* **2011**, *34*, 2515–2520. [CrossRef]
55. Bernasconi, A.A.; Lavie, C.J.; Milani, R.V.; Laukkanen, J.A. Omega-3 Benefits Remain Strong Post-STRENGTH. *Mayo Clin. Proc.* **2021**, *96*, 1371–1372. [CrossRef] [PubMed]
56. Gammelmark, A.; Nielsen, M.S.; Bork, C.S.; Lundbye-Christensen, S.; Tjonneland, A.; Overvad, K.; Schmidt, E.B. Association of fish consumption and dietary intake of marine n-3 PUFA with myocardial infarction in a prospective Danish cohort study. *Br. J. Nutr.* **2016**, *116*, 167–177. [CrossRef] [PubMed]
57. Torris, C.; Molin, M.; Smastuen, M.C. Lean Fish Consumption Is Associated with Beneficial Changes in the Metabolic Syndrome Components: A 13-Year Follow-Up Study from the Norwegian Tromso Study. *Nutrients* **2017**, *9*, 247. [CrossRef]
58. Jakobsen, M.U.; Due, K.M.; Dethlefsen, C.; Halkjaer, J.; Holst, C.; Forouhi, N.G.; Tjonneland, A.; Boeing, H.; Buijsse, B.; Palli, D.; et al. Fish consumption does not prevent increase in waist circumference in European women and men. *Br. J. Nutr.* **2012**, *108*, 924–931. [CrossRef]
59. Bernasconi, A.A.; Wiest, M.M.; Lavie, C.J.; Milani, R.V.; Laukkanen, J.A. Effect of Omega-3 Dosage on Cardiovascular Outcomes: An Updated Meta-Analysis and Meta-Regression of Interventional Trials. *Mayo Clin. Proc.* **2021**, *96*, 304–313. [CrossRef]
60. Okada, L.; Oliveira, C.P.; Stefano, J.T.; Nogueira, M.A.; Silva, I.; Cordeiro, F.B.; Alves, V.A.F.; Torrinhas, R.S.; Carrilho, F.J.; Puri, P.; et al. Omega-3 PUFA modulate lipogenesis, ER stress, and mitochondrial dysfunction markers in NASH—Proteomic and lipidomic insight. *Clin. Nutr.* **2018**, *37*, 1474–1484. [CrossRef]
61. Harris, W.S.; Tintle, N.L.; Imamura, F.; Qian, F.; Korat, A.V.A.; Marklund, M.; Djousse, L.; Bassett, J.K.; Carmichael, P.H.; Chen, Y.Y.; et al. Blood n-3 fatty acid levels and total and cause-specific mortality from 17 prospective studies. *Nat. Commun.* **2021**, *12*, 2329. [CrossRef]
62. Rundblad, A.; Holven, K.B.; Bruheim, I.; Myhrstad, M.C.; Ulven, S.M. Effects of krill oil and lean and fatty fish on cardiovascular risk markers: A randomised controlled trial. *J. Nutr. Sci.* **2018**, *7*, e3. [CrossRef]

63. Kromhout, D.; Giltay, E.J.; Geleijnse, J.M.; Alpha Omega Trial, G. n-3 fatty acids and cardiovascular events after myocardial infarction. *N. Engl. J. Med.* **2010**, *363*, 2015–2026. [CrossRef]
64. Roger, V.L.; Weston, S.A.; Gerber, Y.; Killian, J.M.; Dunlay, S.M.; Jaffe, A.S.; Bell, M.R.; Kors, J.; Yawn, B.P.; Jacobsen, S.J. Trends in incidence, severity, and outcome of hospitalized myocardial infarction. *Circulation* **2010**, *121*, 863–869. [CrossRef]
65. Elagizi, A.; Lavie, C.J.; O'Keefe, E.; Marshall, K.; O'Keefe, J.H.; Milani, R.V. An Update on Omega-3 Polyunsaturated Fatty Acids and Cardiovascular Health. *Nutrients* **2021**, *13*, 204. [CrossRef] [PubMed]
66. Dietary supplementation with n-3 polyunsaturated fatty acids and vitamin E after myocardial infarction: Results of the GISSI-Prevenzione trial. Gruppo Italiano per lo Studio della Sopravvivenza nell'Infarto miocardico. *Lancet* **1999**, *354*, 447–455. [CrossRef]
67. Rauch, B.; Schiele, R.; Schneider, S.; Diller, F.; Victor, N.; Gohlke, H.; Gottwik, M.; Steinbeck, G.; Del Castillo, U.; Sack, R.; et al. OMEGA, a randomized, placebo-controlled trial to test the effect of highly purified omega-3 fatty acids on top of modern guideline-adjusted therapy after myocardial infarction. *Circulation* **2010**, *122*, 2152–2159. [CrossRef] [PubMed]
68. Einvik, G.; Klemsdal, T.O.; Sandvik, L.; Hjerkinn, E.M. A randomized clinical trial on n-3 polyunsaturated fatty acids supplementation and all-cause mortality in elderly men at high cardiovascular risk. *Eur. J. Cardiovasc. Prev. Rehabil.* **2010**, *17*, 588–592. [CrossRef]
69. Samieri, C.; Lorrain, S.; Buaud, B.; Vaysse, C.; Berr, C.; Peuchant, E.; Cunnane, S.C.; Barberger-Gateau, P. Relationship between diet and plasma long-chain n-3 PUFAs in older people: Impact of apolipoprotein E genotype. *J. Lipid Res.* **2013**, *54*, 2559–2567. [CrossRef]
70. Hautero, U.; Poussa, T.; Laitinen, K. Simple dietary criteria to improve serum n-3 fatty acid levels of mothers and their infants. *Public Health Nutr.* **2017**, *20*, 534–541. [CrossRef]
71. Mozaffarian, D.; Wu, J.H. Omega-3 fatty acids and cardiovascular disease: Effects on risk factors, molecular pathways, and clinical events. *J. Am. Coll. Cardiol.* **2011**, *58*, 2047–2067. [CrossRef]
72. Bang, H.Y.; Park, S.A.; Saeidi, S.; Na, H.K.; Surh, Y.J. Docosahexaenoic Acid Induces Expression of Heme Oxygenase-1 and NAD(P)H:quinone Oxidoreductase through Activation of Nrf2 in Human Mammary Epithelial Cells. *Molecules* **2017**, *22*, 969. [CrossRef] [PubMed]
73. Zhu, W.; Ding, Y.; Kong, W.; Li, T.; Chen, H. Docosahexaenoic Acid (DHA) Provides Neuroprotection in Traumatic Brain Injury Models via Activating Nrf2-ARE Signaling. *Inflammation* **2018**, *41*, 1182–1193. [CrossRef] [PubMed]
74. Clarke, S.D. Polyunsaturated fatty acid regulation of gene transcription: A molecular mechanism to improve the metabolic syndrome. *J. Nutr.* **2001**, *131*, 1129–1132. [CrossRef]
75. Jump, D.B. Fatty acid regulation of hepatic lipid metabolism. *Curr. Opin. Clin. Nutr. Metab. Care* **2011**, *14*, 115–120. [CrossRef] [PubMed]
76. de Roos, B.; Mavrommatis, Y.; Brouwer, I.A. Long-chain n-3 polyunsaturated fatty acids: New insights into mechanisms relating to inflammation and coronary heart disease. *Br. J. Pharmacol.* **2009**, *158*, 413–428. [CrossRef] [PubMed]
77. Egert, S.; Stehle, P. Impact of n-3 fatty acids on endothelial function: Results from human interventions studies. *Curr. Opin. Clin. Nutr. Metab. Care* **2011**, *14*, 121–131. [CrossRef]
78. Felau, S.M.; Sales, L.P.; Solis, M.Y.; Hayashi, A.P.; Roschel, H.; Sa-Pinto, A.L.; Andrade, D.C.O.; Katayama, K.Y.; Irigoyen, M.C.; Consolim-Colombo, F.; et al. Omega-3 Fatty Acid Supplementation Improves Endothelial Function in Primary Antiphospholipid Syndrome: A Small-Scale Randomized Double-Blind Placebo-Controlled Trial. *Front. Immunol* **2018**, *9*, 336. [CrossRef]

MDPI
St. Alban-Anlage 66
4052 Basel
Switzerland
Tel. +41 61 683 77 34
Fax +41 61 302 89 18
www.mdpi.com

Nutrients Editorial Office
E-mail: nutrients@mdpi.com
www.mdpi.com/journal/nutrients

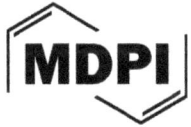

www.ingramcontent.com/pod-product-compliance
Lightning Source LLC
LaVergne TN
LVHW070547100526
838202LV00012B/405